Anti-Wrinkle Treatments for Perfect Skin

48 Recipes for
Masks, Cleansers,
Toners & Lotions
Using Fruit, Herbs
& Other Nourishing
Ingredients

Pierre Jean Cousin

STOREY BOOKS

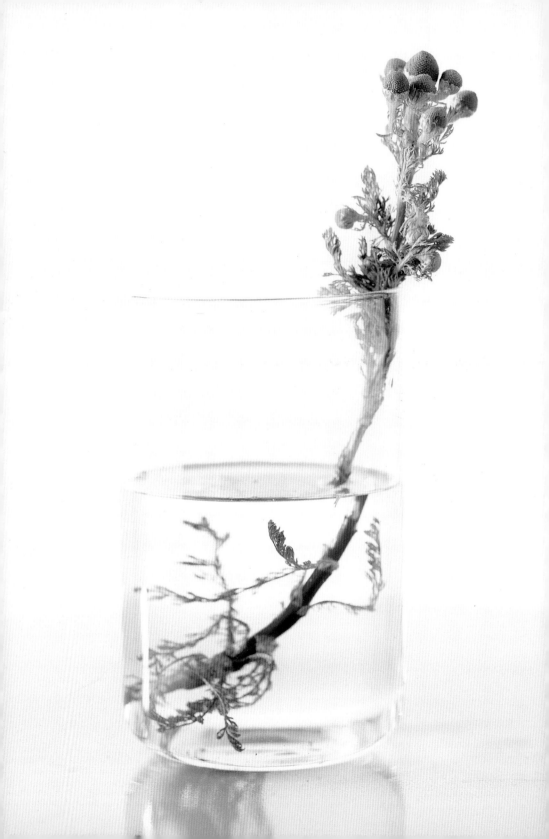

contents

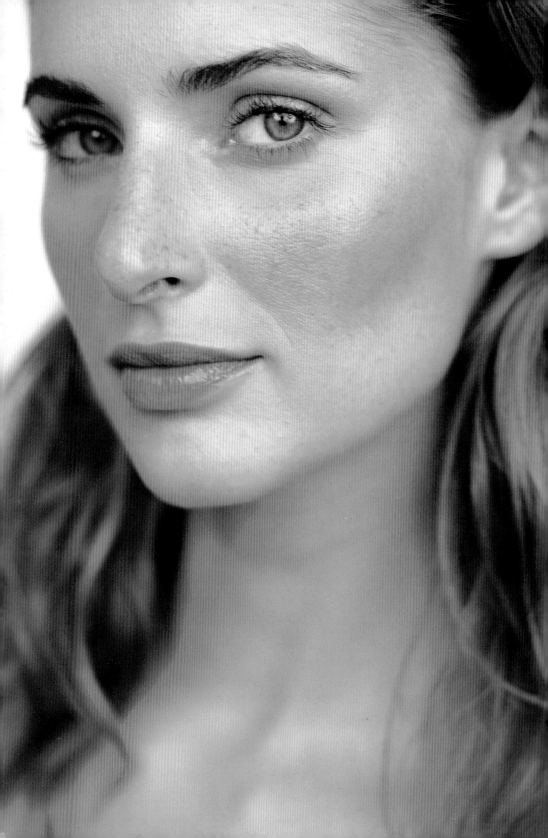

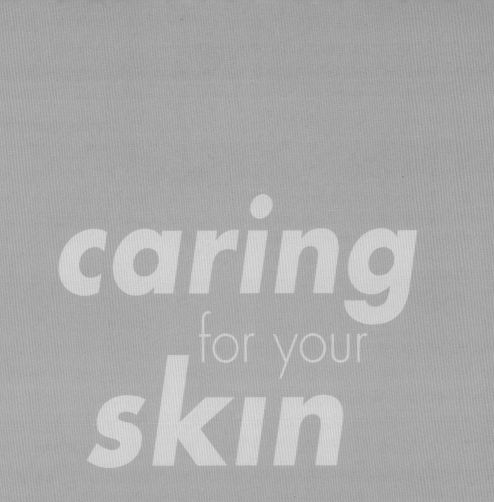

caring for your skin

Look at the skin on any part of your body under a microscope, and it will appear essentially the same. In spite of significant variations due to its particular function, the three layers of epidermis, dermis, and hypodermis will always be visible.

The outer layer, or epidermis, is designed mainly to protect the active layer beneath and to regulate water evaporation. Composed of relatively hardwearing cells, the epidermis is subject to constant renewal as the dead, outermost cells are shed and replaced by new ones. The epidermis contains no blood vessels or nerve endings.

The layer beneath the epidermis, the dermis, is the most hardworking part of the skin and, consequently, the part responsible for most of the aging process of the skin. The multiple functions of the dermis—sensation, thermo-regulation, secretion, and circulation—require a complex structure made up of collagen, elastin, nerve endings, the upper parts of the sebaceous and sweat glands, and small blood vessels (or capillaries). Protein-based collagen fibers team up with elastin to maintain the elasticity of the skin. The greatest concentrations of sebaceous glands occur in the scalp and around the forehead, mouth, and nose, and their main function is to produce sebum, a lubricant indispensable for healthy skin and hair. Sweat glands eliminate toxins and regulate water levels in the body.

Below the dermis is the hypodermis, a layer of connective fatty tissues with a high water content. The hypodermis contains the lower parts of the sebaceous and sweat glands and the hair follicles.

AGING AND THE SKIN
Because we use the skin of the face to monitor changes in temperature and atmospheric conditions, and because we use facial muscle as an important means of expression and communication, facial skin is naturally thinner and more sensitive than the skin on most other parts of our bodies. It is, therefore, on the face that the first signs of aging appear. Yet the inevitable, natural processes of the skin's deterioration, caused by the passing of the years, are at first invisible. By the time we reach adulthood, the life span of our skin cells has shortened dramatically.

The average life of a child's skin cell is 100 days; the average life of an adult's is 50 days.

Between 20 and 25 The earliest visible sign of aging is likely to be the appearance of wrinkles. There are two kinds of wrinkles, and they signal different stages in the aging process. The timing of their appearance is primarily determined by the genetic code, but it is accelerated by, in order of importance, sunlight; smoking; pollution; factors such as wind, dryness, and rapid changes of temperature or humidity; and dietary imbalance. Small, fine, mostly horizontal wrinkles appear first, initially as faint, occasional lines between the eyebrows and at the outer corners of the eyes. These are wrinkles of expression, and they are accentuated by laughing. Light freckles, if present, indicate over-exposure to the sun; they increase in number during the summer months.

Between 25 and 35 More horizontal superficial lines of expression become visible on the forehead and possibly around the mouth. The first lowering wrinkles may also appear—faint vertical lines between the outer edges of the nostrils and the corners of the mouth. These are the result of changes taking place in the hypodermis, as gravity causes the fatty cells to migrate downward. There is also a slight softening of the skin of the neck; it is beginning to lose its tone. Small, irregular, brown patches may appear as the skin pigments react to sudden over-exposure to sunlight.

By 40 Very gradually, the wrinkles of expression and lowering become deeper and more permanent. Lack of skin tone in the neck increases, creating "necklaces" of criss-crossing horizontal lines. The hypodermis of the neck has fewer fat cells and fewer of the sebaceous glands necessary to keep the skin hydrated. Without adequate moisture, the skin of the neck is particularly vulnerable to the effects of aging.

Between 45 and 55 By 45, facial contours begin to change as the bones thin and the skin loses some of its elasticity due to the disappearance of elastin in the dermis. In many cases, the collagen is still intact, but the skin has become softer and dryer. The ability of the skin to retain water is greatly diminished—by up to one-third if you compare the skin of a child with that of a mature adult. After the age of 45, the rate of aging increases. The epidermis becomes thinner and, as the elastin continues to disappear, the collagen structure is disrupted, causing the dermo–epidermis to flatten. This is often vastly accelerated by lifestyle, in particular by smoking and prolonged exposure to sun. Changes in the hypodermis also speed up as the distribution of fatty tissues and fluid becomes more uneven, and the effects of gravity increase the lowering process.

Between 55 and 65 A significant lowering of fatty tissues toward the chin and the lower jaw may change the shape of the face. Skin texture thickens on the face and neck. The disruption of collagen continues, and the cells responsible for the restoration of elastin in the dermis disappear altogether.

After 65 As structural changes occur in the skin, the skin's functions are also altered. The healing process takes longer, bruising becomes more frequent, waste products are eliminated more slowly, sensitivity is reduced, and blood circulation is less efficient. In time, the skin becomes more sensitive to infections and, finally, production of vitamin D and protection against the sun are impaired.

Aging may be a genetically determined, essentially irreversible process that can be accelerated by chronic illnesses, such as diabetes and atherosclerosis, but it is important to eliminate any aggravating factors as far as possible to maintain and preserve the integrity of the three layers of the skin, both structurally and functionally.

Stress, pollution, and changes in hormonal balance can all contribute to the premature aging of the skin, but recent research shows that regular smokers invariably age far more quickly than non-smokers age. The damage is done in the dermis. The elastin and collagen deteriorate faster, and vital supplies of oxygen and nutrients are reduced as nicotine contracts the capillaries to create gray, lifeless skin. Today, however, the skin's greatest enemy of all is the sun.

SUN AND THE SKIN

The most important external factor in the aging of the skin is over-exposure to the harmful rays of the sun. Some exposure to sunlight is beneficial—it stimulates the production of vitamin D, a substance essential for the formation and maintenance of healthy bones—but regular, prolonged sunbathing and exposure to ultraviolet rays can be very destructive. The dangers have increased considerably in recent years as a result of the destruction of the ozone layer.

There are two types of ultraviolet rays. Ultraviolet B short-wave rays burn the two outer layers of the skin. Only 10 percent of UVB rays reach the dermis, but they act upon the collagen–elastin association, causing its rapid and premature dissociation and a significant loss of elasticity. Strongest at low latitudes and high altitudes, ultraviolet A long-wave rays are known to penetrate more deeply into the skin, contributing even more to the processes of wrinkling and loss of elasticity that result in aging. Although UVB rays are thought to be responsible for sunburn and most skin cancers—more than 90 percent of U.S. skin cancers are attributed to UVB exposure—it is possible that UVA rays play some part in the causes of skin cancer.

Almost all sunscreens protect against UVB rays, but nothing is available to screen out all UVA rays. Even sunscreens offering a high sun protection factor (SPF)—a standard designed to measure a sunscreen's ability to protect the skin and prevent sunburn—leave your skin vulnerable to damage from UVA rays. Some researchers estimate that sunscreens advertising UVA protection actually offer only SPF3 or 4 protection against UVA rays; the higher stated SPF figure relates only to protection against UVB rays.

CHOOSING A SUNSCREEN

Of course, people burn at different rates, even within the same skin type, so you must decide if you are more or less sensitive to sun exposure and take appropriate measures. Information about the dangers of sun exposure is now widely available. Wear clothing that covers the body and shades the face. Apply an appropriate sunscreen to all exposed areas of the body, reapplying every two hours, even on cloudy days, and after swimming or perspiring. Minimize sun exposure between 10 a.m. and 3 p.m. Avoid unnecessary exposure to radiation from sun

skin color	risk of freckles	risk of sunburn	tan type	recommended minimum protection
albino	○	•••••	none; red sunburn with pain, swelling and peeling	SPF50
white	•••••	••••	as above	SPF50
fair	••••	•••	very light after minor pink or red burns	SPF30–50
fair	•••	••	light	SPF30
slightly dark	○	••	dark	SPF30
slightly dark	○	•	dark	SPF15–20
dark	○	○	very dark	SPF8–15
black	○	○	black	SPF8

••••• = maximum risk   ○ = minimum risk

lamps or tanning parlors. These precautions are necessary to protect the skin against an increasing risk of skin cancer as well as premature aging.

The table above indicates general guidelines for minimum protection. To be on the safe side, always reduce by half the stated protection on any product. In reality, a cream labeled SPF8, for example, may for certain types of skin and in particular external conditions (such as wind, salt water, or heavy perspiration) offer only SPF4 protection. Be aware that a tan is little protection from skin damage—it is reckoned to be equal to SPF2.

SKIN TYPES

The first step in any personal natural skin-care program is to establish which skin type you have. There are five basic groups, and a simple tissue test (see page 12) will establish which one is yours. It is worth doing this test even if you are confident of the result. Health, time, environment, and even season can cause temporary or permanent changes in skin condition. In fact, it is worth repeating the test every six months.

Normal skin Firm, supple, warm to the touch, neither dry nor greasy, and without spots or blemishes—it is easiest to care for this type of skin. Normal skin is neither too acid nor too alkaline, with an average, neutral pH of 6.5.

Dry skin Often slightly hot to the touch, dry skin is prone to powdery scaling, superficial wrinkling, and a dull appearance. This more acid skin type is sensitive to cold and wind and to central heating and to air conditioning. It rapidly becomes irritated and inflamed, requiring regular applications of moisturizer.

Oily skin Frequent pimples and small inflamed areas are a reality with oily skin, which is prone to acne and dermatitis. Excess sebum (see page 6) leaves oily skin with a neglected appearance, making it shiny and difficult to keep clean. Sun; alcohol; poor diet; stress; and cold, damp winters aggravate the effects. Sebum inhibits water loss, so this alkaline type can age slowly.

Combination skin Dry with shiny, oily areas on the forehead, sides of the nose, and around the mouth and chin, combination skin is difficult to care for because some areas need deep moisturizing while others need astringent, drying applications.

Aging skin Tending towards dryness, aging skin is often hot to the touch and sometimes blemished, damaged, or flushed with erythema (a hereditary redness due to the dilation of capillaries in the dermis). It lacks tone and flexibility—a simple pinch will indicate how quickly it recovers. Aging skin needs constant attention with toner, hydrating lotions, and nourishing masks.

Two other skin types will be mentioned frequently in this book: sensitive skin and damaged skin. The term sensitive skin is used to describe any skin type that responds especially quickly and adversely to sudden changes of temperature or humidity and bruises very easily. Sensitive skin is also allergic to many cosmetic products. It demands constant attention (see the special program on page 19). Damaged skin usually describes a localized area of skin with a texture and/or appearance that has changed because of a condition, such as acne or eczema. Whether it is dry, oily, or combination skin, damaged skin will exhibit some inflammation, scaling, thickening, or scarring. Special care is needed for these areas (see page 120).

THE TISSUE TEST

You need a completely clean face for this, so remove any traces of makeup and give your face a final cleaning, using warm water and cotton pads. Gently towel dry and wait for about 30 minutes before covering your face with one ply (or layer) of a family-size paper tissue. Press lightly all over your face and leave for about 1 minute. Then remove the tissue carefully and examine it near a window or a light.

Normal skin Faint oily traces on most of the paper.

Dry skin No oily traces—very often aging skin is dry.

Oily skin Clear oily stains over most of the paper.

Combination skin Oily patches at the sides of the nose and around the mouth and forehead.

BASIC SKIN CARE

The three important aspects of skin maintenance are well known, and it is never too early to begin. Indeed, teenagers need to pay particular attention to their skin. A mild condition—a few spots, a small rash, or eczema—can, if neglected, become severe, leading to scarring.

Cleansing Good cleansing removes the impurities, bacteria, and dead cells that accumulate on the surface of the epidermis, as well as any makeup residue, while leaving as much of the lubricating natural oil (or sebum) as possible. A cleanser should, therefore, be gentle and natural. Unless your face is covered with mechanic's grease, there's no benefit in scrubbing with detergents and water: Harsh detergent soaps and rubbing only strip the skin of vital oils and nutrients. A lotion is usually enough for daily cleansing. Once in a while, or on a more regular basis for those with oily skin, a clay, fruit, or oat cleansing mask or some steaming should be used for a much deeper cleansing action.

Nourishing Dry and aging skin in particular need additional hydration and oily substances, as well as minerals and small amounts of essential vitamins, to help maintain and regenerate normal vitality.

Toning Again, toning is particularly important in maintaining the elasticity of dry and aging skin. However, it is vital to hydrate at the same time in order to maintain a normal level of fluid in the skin. It is for this reason that the natural toning recipes in this book combine astringents (to close the pores and reduce water loss) and moistening agents.

Some conventional skin-care programs may present those three vital steps in a different order: cleanse, tone, and then nourish. Natural-care programs are based on the belief that it makes sense to close the pores *after* you feed the skin. So, anyone who needs to nourish, should remember the best routine: It's cleanse, nourish, and then tone.

STARTING THE NATURAL SKIN-CARE PROGRAM

Any of the recipes given in this book will fulfill at least one of these three tasks. Most of them offer a combination of beneficial actions. Once you have determined your skin type, you are ready to explore the recipe chapters. The summary at the foot of each recipe indicates the principal effects and appropriate skin types at a glance. Read about basic techniques in the next chapter, which includes a section on massage and the application of essential oils (see pages 20–47) and other recipes to try.

All the recipes are easy to prepare, but to make the most of them you must apply them at regular intervals in a coherent program. The following pages set out programs for each of the five basic skin types and for those with sensitive skin. The book ends with a section devoted to common skin conditions, where there are recommended programs and additional recipes. Once you have established a workable and successful maintenance routine, experiment by introducing other appropriate recipes and treatments—one at a time. You'll soon discover what works for you.

normal skin

teens

Use a gentle cleanser, such as a chamomile infusion (see page 30), daily. A cleansing or nourishing clay, fruit (not too strong—avoid those containing citrus juices, papaya, strawberry, or tomato), or oat mask can be applied once every two weeks to eliminate dead cells and promote regeneration. In summer or after exposure to wind, use herbal hydrating ice cubes (see page 32).
Hydrosols: chamomile, cornflower, lavender, orange blossom, rose, rosemary.

20s to 30s

See "teens" for cleansing, mask routine, and herbal ice cubes. Begin to introduce recipes containing hydrating or toning ingredients, such as honey and cucumber milk (see page 54), or rose, honey, and lemon lotion (see page 111). Apple cider vinegar (see page 46) is also good.
Essential oils: chamomile, geranium, lavender, niaouli, palmarosa, rosemary, rose otto, rosewood.
Carrier oils: hazelnut, olive, sweet almond.
Hydrosols: see "teens."

30s to 40s

Use a gentle cleanser containing hydrating and balancing ingredients daily (see "teens" and "20s to 30s") and follow with a mild toner, such as rose hydrosol and witch hazel cleanser (see page 62), apple cologne (see page 104), or rose hydrosol astringent lotion (see page 106). Massage face and neck once a day with a suitable oil mix (see pages 34–44). Choose a cleansing and toning mask containing citrus juice (orange, grapefruit, or lemon), dairy products, or honey, and use once a week.
Essential oils: see "20s to 30s."
Carrier oils: see "20s to 30s," plus apricot kernel, lime (or linden) blossom, wheat germ.
Hydrosols: see "teens."

40s to 50s

See "30s to 40s" for daily routine with cleanser, toner, and massage. Once a week, alternate a series of toning and nourishing masks and lotions. Avoid exfoliating ingredients, such as papaya or tomato, which may now be too harsh, putting emphasis on nourishing recipes containing borage oil, evening primrose oil, wheat germ oil, or vitamin E oil.
Essential oils: see "20s to 30s," substituting clary sage, cypress, frankincense for niaouli.
Carrier oils: see "20s to 30s," plus macadamia nut.
Hydrosols: chamomile, clary sage, rosemary, rose, witch hazel.

50s+

See section on aging skin (page 18).

dry skin

teens

Use a gentle cleanser, such as almond milk (see page 50), daily. Avoid steaming, but compresses or herbal ice cubes (see pages 30–32) can be used at any time. Alternate hydrating blackcurrant and nourishing banana fruit masks—use one once a week. An oatmeal and lemon juice mask (see page 67) can be used once every two weeks to remove dead cells. The yogurt and carrot juice mask (see page 76) is also an excellent way to nourish the skin and maintain a good pH. Experiment with the clay and cucumber recipe (see page 55), adding 2 tablespoons of olive or sweet almond oil. Massage face and neck once a day with a suitable oil mix (see pages 34–44).

Essential oils: chamomile, geranium, lavender, palmarosa, rosemary, rose otto, rosewood.

Carrier oils: olive, sweet almond.

Hydrosols: orange blossom (neroli), rose, rosemary.

20s to 30s

See "teens." The honey and cucumber cleansing milk (see page 54) is another gentle cleanser that can be used daily.

Essential oils: see "teens," plus frankincense, orange blossom (neroli).

Carrier oils: apricot kernel, macadamia nut, olive, wheat germ.

Hydrosols: clary sage, rosemary, rose.

30s to 40s

See "teens" and "20s to 30s" for daily cleansing and see advice on steaming (page 33), compresses (pages 32–33), ice cubes (page 32), and massage (pages 42–44). Alternate nourishing, hydrating, and toning masks containing avocado, banana, blackcurrant, and grape as appropriate once a week. A simple oatmeal mask with an added teaspoon of lemon juice (see page 27) can be used occasionally to eliminate dead cells, tone, and promote regeneration. The spirulina mask (see page 74) and the healing mask (see page 89) are also excellent for nourishing and revitalizing the skin. Experiment with any recipe that combines ingredients that nourish (honey and cream) with those that tone (lemon and egg white).

Essential oils: see "teens" and "20s to 30s," omitting lavender.

Carrier oils: see "20s to 30s," plus borage.

Hydrosols: see "20s to 30s," plus chamomile, cornflower, witch hazel.

40s to 50s

See section on aging skin (page 18).

50s+

See section on aging skin (page 18).

oily skin

teens

Use daily a simple cleansing lotion such as rose hydrosol and lemon juice (see page 59) or a chamomile infusion (see page 30). That, and steaming (see page 33) once a week, may be all that is needed to prevent clogged pores, inflammation, and fatty deposits under the skin. Once every one or two weeks, apply a clay mask made with cucumber juice (see page 55) or a chamomile infusion, (see page 30) and no more than once a month try a clay mask using citrus juice or a fruit mask containing raspberry or tomato. Apple cider vinegar (see page 46) is also helpful. Massage face and neck once a day with a suitable oil mix (see pages 34–44).

Essential oils: cedarwood, chamomile, cypress, juniper, lavender, lemon, mandarin, patchouli, rosewood.

Carrier oils: calendula, hazelnut, hypericum (St. John's wort), jojoba, olive, sweet almond.

Hydrosols: chamomile, lavender, orange blossom (neroli), rose.

20s to 30s

See "teens." For deeper cleansing, use the pineapple (see page 65) or papaya exfoliators (see page 68) to remove blackheads and spots.

Essential oils, carrier oils and hydrosols: see "teens."

30s to 40s

See "teens" and "20s to 30s."

Essential oils: see "teens." Also niaouli and tea tree.

Carrier oils and hydrosols: see "teens."

40s to 50s

Even oily skin tends to become dry with time. Use a gentle cleanser, such as almond (see page 50) or honey and cucumber milk (see page 54), daily, and massage. Steam once every two weeks (see page 33); but compresses or ice cubes (see pages 30–32) can be used at any time. Try the clay and cucumber cleansing mask (see page 55), adding 1 tablespoon of borage oil. Use a nourishing banana or hydrating blackcurrant fruit mask once a week, plus an oatmeal mask with lemon juice (see page 27) every 2–3 weeks to promote regeneration. Experiment with toners, and recipes using yogurt, cream, or honey.

Essential oils: chamomile, clary sage, cypress, frankincense, geranium, lavender, lemon, myrrh, rosemary, rose otto, rosewood.

Carrier oils: apricot kernel, macadamia nut, olive, wheat germ.

Hydrosols: chamomile, clary sage, cornflower, orange blossom (neroli), rosemary, rose.

50s+

See section on aging skin (page 18).

combination skin

Steam (see page 33) once a week to check oily areas, but use a gentle cleanser, such as almond milk (see page 50), or a chamomile infusion (see page 30), daily. Once every 1–2 weeks, apply a clay mask made with cucumber juice (see page 55) or chamomile infusion, and once a month a clay mask, using orange or grapefruit juice, or a raspberry or tomato fruit mask. Massage face and neck once a day with a suitable oil mix (see pages 34–44).

Essential oils: cedarwood, chamomile, cypress, lavender, lemon, mandarin, orange blossom (neroli), patchouli, rosewood, tea tree.

Carrier oils: calendula, hazelnut, hypericum, jojoba, olive, sweet almond.

Hydrosols: chamomile, lavender, orange blossom (neroli), rose.

Using almond milk (see page 50), rose hydrosol and lemon juice (see page 59), or clay milk (see page 58), cleanse the face daily. Steam once a week (see page 33) and apply a clay mask using carrot juice, not water (see pages 22–24), or try a yogurt- or oat-based mask. Apply a clay and citrus-juice mask or fruit mask (see "teens") every 2–3 weeks. Apple cider (see page 46) is also useful.

Essential oils, carrier oils and hydrosols: see "teens."

For steaming, daily cleansing, massage, fruit masks, and apple cider vinegar, see "20s to 30s," minus the cleansing milk. Once a week, apply a clay mask made with carrot juice (see pages 22–24) or geranium oil (see page 73), or apply a yogurt- or oatmeal-based mask. Consider regular use of a toning mask or lotion, such as barley and rosemary lotion (see page 108), fresh juice toner (see page 110), or yogurt and blackcurrant mask (see page 99).

Essential oils, carrier oils and hydrosols: see "teens."

Combination skin tends to become dry now. For daily cleansing, massage, and apple cider vinegar, see "20s to 30s." For a once-weekly mask, see "30s to 40s." Every 2–3 weeks try an extra-nourishing clay mask, adding 2 tablespoons of chopped parsley to the mix (see page 23), or the spirulina vitalizing mask (see page 74). For regular toning, see "30s to 40s."

Essential oils: see "teens," substituting clary sage, frankincense, geranium, for mandarin.

Carrier oils: see "teens," plus borage.

Hydrosols: see "teens," plus clary sage.

See section on aging skin (page 18).

aging skin

30s to 40s

Constant nourishing and toning is essential for skin showing signs of premature aging. Use an astringent and toning cleanser, such as rose hydrosol and lemon juice (see page 59) or rose hydrosol and witch hazel (see page 62), daily. Twice a week, enjoy a nourishing mask, such as the spirulina vitalizing mask (see page 74), banana anti-aging mask (see page 72), high nutrient and vitamin mask (see page 88) or almond and egg white mask (see page 81). If possible, apply a toner, such as fresh juice toner (see page 110) or cucumber and vinegar lotion (see page 107), or one of the toning and hydrating masks, daily. Use apple cider vinegar (see page 46) when washing your face or in the bath. Daily massage and the application of essential oils becomes an even more important part of the fight against dehydration (see pages 34–44).

Essential oils: cedarwood, chamomile, clary sage, cypress, frankincense, geranium, lavender, myrrh, palmarosa, rose otto, rosewood, sandalwood.

Carrier oils: apricot kernel, borage, evening primrose, hazelnut, hypericum, lime (or linden) blossom, macadamia nut, olive, rosehip seed, wheat germ.

Hydrosols: chamomile, clary sage, cornflower, orange blossom (neroli), rose.

40s to 50s

See "30s to 40s."

Essential oils, carrier oils and hydrosols: see "30s to 40s."

50s+

See "30s to 40s." The oil mixture for daily massage should be a prepared blend of 3½ tablespoons (50ml) rosehip seed and 3½ tablespoons (50ml) lime (or linden) blossom as joint carriers (if unavailable, use hypericum or olive) plus ⅖ teaspoon (2ml) clary sage, ⅕ teaspoon (1ml) geranium, ⅕ teaspoon (1ml) frankincense and ⅕ teaspoon (1ml) sandalwood essential oils (see pages 34–44).

Essential oils, carrier oils and hydrosols: see "30s to 40s."

sensitive skin

teens

Use a chamomile tea (see page 30) daily as a face wash, followed by the traditional almond milk (see page 50) or honey and cucumber cleansing milk (see page 54). The hydrosols listed below can be used as often as you like (see also page 45). Make an oil mix, using olive oil as a carrier with a blend of lavender, rosewood, and tea tree, and massage the face and neck once a day (see pages 34–44). Avoid any treatment that may be too harsh for sensitive skin, such as masks containing strawberry, tomato, or papaya, but once every two weeks use an oatmeal and lemon mask, substituting a chamomile infusion for the witch hazel (see page 67). Use apple cider vinegar (see page 46) when washing your face or in the bath.

Essential oils: cedarwood, chamomile, cypress, lavender, lemon, rosewood, tea tree.

Carrier oils: calendula, hazelnut, olive, sweet almond.

Hydrosols: chamomile, cornflower, lavender, orange blossom (neroli), rose.

20s to 30s

See "teens." Alternate the mask you apply once every two weeks, using the oatmeal and lemon mask with a chamomile infusion (see page 67, VARIATIONS), light nourishing masks such as yogurt and carrot juice (see page 76), or the toning yogurt and blackcurrant (see page 99).

Essential oils: see "teens." Also frankincense.

Carrier oils: see "teens."

Hydrosols: see "teens."

30s to 40s

See "teens," adding the alternative masks under "20s to 30s." An astringent and toning cleanser, such as rose hydrosol and lemon juice (see page 59), can also be used every day.

Essential oils: see "teens." Also frankincense.

Carrier oils: see "teens." Also borage or evening primrose.

Hydrosols: see "teens."

40s to 50s

See section on aging skin (page 18).

50s+

See section on aging skin (page 18).

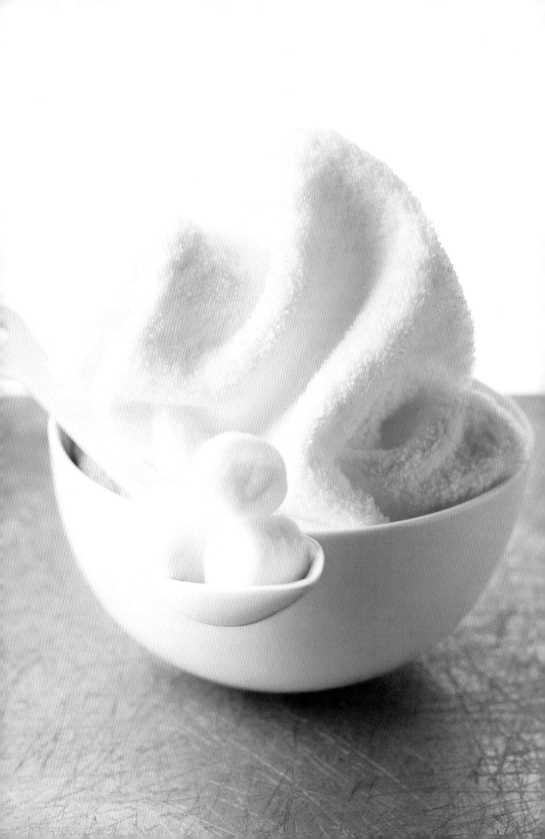

basic
techniques

masks and lotions

The masks and lotions in this book offer all the basic tools you need for short- and long-term natural skin care. Obtaining your skin products from simple, seasonal, raw ingredients means that you have immediate and direct access to a complex mixture of natural substances far more beneficial to your skin than the synthetic counterparts used in many of today's commercial cosmetics. And, because these recipes are so inexpensive and simple to make, you have the opportunity to build a skin-care program that responds week by week, season by season, to the current state of your skin, whatever your environment.

clay

Clay is an immensely versatile ingredient in skin care. As a deep cleanser, it detoxifies by drawing impurities out from beneath the epidermis. As a nourisher, it contributes trace elements important to the maintenance of healthy skin. As a toner, its astringent action is best associated with ingredients, such as lemon juice or hydrosol (see page 45). Therapeutically, clay is also antiseptic, anti-inflammatory, and analgesic.

TYPES OF CLAY

A sediment formed by the slow erosion of granite, clay contains various minerals, such as iron oxide, salts, calcium, and other trace elements in varying proportions that alter its color and therapeutic qualities. Three kinds are commonly available for cosmetic purposes.

White clay (or kaolin) is rich in silica and magnesium. This clay is neutral and not too drying, and it is effective in absorbing impurities and putting valuable minerals back into the skin. It is suitable for all types of skin (especially dry skin) as a mask or lotion. Green clay (or montmorillonite) brings more mineral and trace elements to the skin, being rich in silica, manganese, potassium, aluminum, and iron oxide, but it is also more drying. Its powerful action is most suitable for problem skin conditions, including acne, seborrhoea, eczema, or damaged skin. Red clay (also montmorillonite, or sometimes illite or attapulgite) has properties and indications similar to those of green clay. Its red color is due to a high concentration of iron oxide.

Cosmetic clay is available in three forms, apart from the ready-made masks sold at greatly inflated prices. You may find it in an enterprising supermarket, but there are a number of specialty suppliers (see page 126). Buy it in powder form if you can. Clay powder is easy to use, absorbing water or any other liquid rapidly and mixing well with other solid ingredients, such as blue-green algae (also called spirulina), chopped herbs, or puréed fruit or vegetables. Clay is also sold as a paste, ready to use. Although this is clearly timesaving, it does limit the sort of mask you can make because some recipes require that other ingredients be added to the clay before the liquid. It is also more expensive.

MAKING A CLAY MASK

The method of making a basic clay mask is very simple. The required amount of clay (usually 2–3 tablespoons) is just covered with bottled or spring water (the water should settle about 5mm above the clay) and left to rest for a minimum of 30 minutes without stirring. Water that is low on minerals is recommended; do not use tap water or any water that contains chlorine. It is important not to stir until after the resting period (when all the water has been absorbed) because premature stirring affects the consistency of the mask, making it sticky and lumpy and, therefore, more difficult to apply.

Once the resting period is over, stir the ingredients thoroughly to mix well. To be ready to use, the mixture must have the consistency of a thick paste that can be applied with ease. If it is too liquid, it will not adhere, and if it is too thick, it will not penetrate deeply into the skin. It is easy enough to add a small amount of clay to a mix that is too thin, but adding more water to a paste that is too thick requires great care: add very gradually, stirring all the time.

If other ingredients are to be added to the clay, it is preferable to do so at this stage, but any oil or blend of oils (see page 37) is best added to the dry clay. Some of the recipes in this book substitute fruit or vegetable juices or hydrosols for bottled or spring water. The same rules on resting and stirring apply. Clay powder (or oat flour) is also used as a thickening agent in some lighter masks. No resting time is necessary in most cases—follow the recipe instructions. To be effective, a clay mask is best applied at least once or twice a week. See pages 27–29 for how to make the most of a clay mask, including application and removal.

fruit

Many of the fruits we eat every day make excellent masks that have a revitalizing, nourishing, and often astringent action on the skin. It is the variety of acids they contain (including malic, glycolic, citric, salicylic, and tartric acid) and their high vitamin and mineral content that bring these benefits.

Indeed, fruit acids are now extracted (alpha-hydroxy acids) or chemically synthesized (beta-hydroxy acids) commercially and used by cosmetic surgeons as chemical peeling agents at high concentrations for those prepared to suffer pain and risk burns, allergic reactions, and hypersensitization to the sun in pursuit of a more youthful appearance.

Fortunately, the natural ingredients in simple fruit masks—in which the crushed flesh or juice of fresh fruits is applied directly to the skin—have a milder action, acting in synergy without dangerous side effects. All the fruit masks given in this book can be applied frequently and are beneficial in many ways for a variety of skin types, especially for those with dry or aging skin.

The gentle peeling action of a fruit mask removes dead skin, excess fatty deposits, and blackheads from the epidermis; eliminates freckles and excess pigmentation; and erases faint lines and wrinkles of expression. By increasing acidity on the surface of the skin, a fruit mask also inhibits the growth of bacteria, helps regulate the secretion of sebum, unclogs and closes pores, and tones and hydrates the skin. In addition, a fruit mask contributes small amounts of trace elements and minerals essential for healthy skin, such as potassium, zinc, and selenium.

However, there is one warning note to sound for anyone who has sensitive skin or is potentially allergic. It is not wise to use highly acidic fruit masks (such as those containing tomatoes) more than once a week. Test for possible allergic reactions on a small portion of the skin on the inside arm. Apply a small amount of the fruit mask directly to the skin, leave on for 2–3 minutes, remove with a cotton pad, wait another 10 minutes, and then check for any redness where the mask was applied.

USING FRUIT FOR MASKS AND LOTIONS

The best fruits to use for cleansing, toning, and nourishing are apple, apricot, avocado, banana, blackcurrant, cherry, grape, grapefruit, lemon, melon, orange, raspberry, papaya, pineapple, and tomato. Use the freshest fruit you can find, preferably organically grown, and if a recipe requires fruit juices, make them yourself whenever possible, again using fresh ingredients. Fresh carrot and grape juice are acceptable as long as they are sold in a carton, but avoid long-life, UHT (ultra high temperature), and canned products.

Most fruit masks and lotions are extremely easy to make, either by hand or by using a food processor or blender. The fruit is crushed to a purée or its juice is extracted, and the resulting product is simply and speedily mixed with other natural ingredients, such as dairy products, honey, eggs, hydrosols (see page 45), or oils (see pages 34–41). If the consistency of a purée needs a bulking agent to make a mask that can be easily applied, a small amount of clay powder, oatmeal, oat flour, or yogurt with live and active cultures is often added, without compromising the benefits of the purée. Juices from fruits such as grapefruit, lemon, orange, grape, or tomato are also mixed with larger amounts of clay or stiffly beaten egg white to create an effective mask, or applied directly to the skin as a lotion, either alone or in association with other natural ingredients. See pages 27–29 for how to make the most of masks and lotions.

vegetables

Masks based on fresh vegetable ingredients have useful anti-inflammatory action, making them a must for sensitive, damaged, or inflamed skin. In addition to having cooling properties, they promote healing by giving the damaged epidermis large amounts of vitamin A, important minerals, and trace elements. For this reason, vegetable masks are most valuable at times of crisis — sudden outbreaks of acne or eczema, sunburn, and allergic reactions to food or medical drugs — although they are good for cleansing and nourishing, too.

USING VEGETABLES FOR MASKS AND LOTIONS

The most valuable vegetables for skin care are cabbage, carrot, cucumber, lettuce, potato, and watercress. The herb parsley is also beneficial. Always use the freshest possible ingredients, organically grown if available, and make your own juice whenever possible.

There are many simple ways to include vegetables in your skin care program. Cucumber (grated or juiced) can be added to clay for a number of effective masks, and cucumber or carrot juice can be applied directly to the skin, in association with other ingredients, as a lotion. Fresh parsley or watercress can simply be chopped and added to a clay mask, yogurt with live and active cultures, or heavy cream. The green vegetables — lettuce, watercress, or cabbage — can be puréed and then thickened with clay or oatmeal to apply as a mask. Alternatively, the cooked and cooled leaves of lettuce or cabbage can be applied directly to the skin, and the cooking water can be used as a gentle lotion. Oat flour (or clay) is also used as a bulking agent in some lighter masks. See pages 27–29 for how to make the most of masks and lotions.

other ingredients

Barley In the recipes in this book, only barley water is used, in a lotion, but cooked barley can be processed into a paste and used as a mask.
Dairy Whole milk and yogurt with live and active cultures are used to balance and cleanse, whereas cream (and it must be thick, heavy

cream) adds nourishment. Thickener is essential in any dairy-based mask. See "eggs" for advice on storage.

Eggs Yolks are added to masks to make them more nourishing and to thicken; stiffly beaten whites make a mask more astringent and adhesive and easier to spread. Masks containing egg must be used quickly, although they can be stored for up to 6 hours in a refrigerator.

Honey Usually added to other substances such as clay, eggs, fruit, or yogurt, honey enhances the nourishing qualities of a mask or a lotion. It also acts as a thickening and "adhesive" agent.

Oats Oatmeal and oatbran can be used cooked or raw as the basis of a mask. Cooked in water and cooled, they can be used as a mask. Uncooked, they can be bound with water (sometimes with 1 teaspoon of lemon juice) or with milk or yogurt; in this state they are often extremely absorbent. Oatmeal is also an excellent thickener.

Pollen A teaspoon of powdered or ground pollen enriches any mask and is very useful for aging or damaged skin. Add a little more liquid—fruit juice, water, or hydrosol—as the recipe dictates.

Royal jelly Because of its creamy consistency, royal jelly can be added to a mask without further adjustment, just before the mask is applied.

IMPORTANT: BEFORE YOU MAKE A MASK

Most metals oxidize when in contact with clay and fruit or vegetable juices, so avoid using metal mixing bowls or containers. Similarly, do not use a metal spoon or spatula for stirring, although the stainless-steel blades of a processor or blender are fine. Make sure that all equipment is absolutely clean. The quantities indicated for some of the recipes may vary according to the quality of the ingredients, or according to the weather. In dry, hot weather, for example, you may need to add more liquid. It is assumed that you are using a small blender or processor; there is inevitably more wastage with family size models, and you may have to double quantities. Warm water may be used when making a mask, but never heat a mask. Don't be tempted to save time by making large quantities. Masks are best made just before they are used, although the recipes specify shelf life.

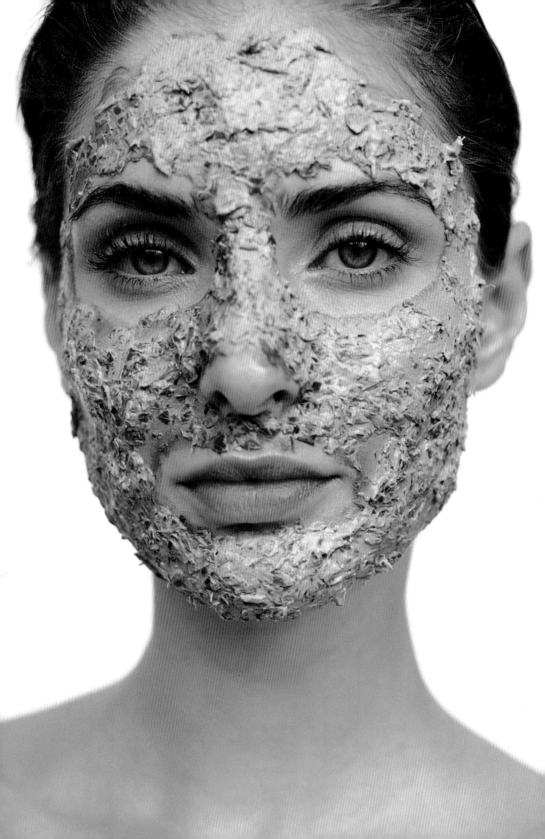

applying masks and lotions

The following sequence sets out the ideal process of using a natural mask or lotion. Unfortunately, many of us today lead such busy lives that we find it difficult to devote this much time to ourselves. Aim to find that time maybe once a week and, when that is not possible, skip step 4 and maybe combine steps 2 and 3.

1 Find a quiet, calm time and place. When you allow yourself the space to slow down and enjoy the simple processes of preparing, applying, and removing a mask, you are likely to be more centered, and that means more receptive and responsive.

2 Put on a headband to protect your hair, and remove any makeup. Then carefully clean the skin with cotton pads and bottled or spring water; an herbal infusion (see page 30), using chamomile, rosemary, or lavender flowers; a hydrosol (see page 45); or one of the simpler cleansing recipes (see pages 50 and 59).

3 Relax your facial muscles in any way that suits you. It might be by using massage or by making hideous faces at yourself in the mirror.

4 Steam your face gently (1–2 minutes over a bowl of hot water) or apply a hot compress for 2 minutes (see pages 33 and 32). Both techniques open the pores so that the mask can penetrate more deeply.

5 Apply the mask evenly, avoiding the area around the eyes (unless, of course, it is an eye mask) and using your fingers or cotton pads as appropriate. Fruit or egg masks often have a very liquid consistency. It may be easier to apply a second layer after a few minutes, once the first layer has dried a little.

6 Try not to talk, laugh, or move any facial muscle until it is time to gently remove the mask.

7 Remove the mask slowly and carefully. Work from the forehead downward, making sure that none of the material removed comes into contact with the eyes, and avoid dragging the skin. Light fruit masks can be removed simply with cotton pads. With clay masks, you need to rinse the face first to soften the clay.

8 Where appropriate, spray or apply a hydrosol to close the pores and tone the skin. See the recipes and the listings on pages 14–19 for guidance.

herbal infusions

Fresh and dried herbs have been used to make infusions with medical properties, applied externally or used with compresses, for thousands of years. The list below outlines the properties and benefits of the principal herbs recommended for use in herbal infusions. Several have cleansing and toning qualities that make them useful in any long-term natural skin-care program; all are suitable for any type of skin.

Calendula (marigold flower) Use healing calendula alone or in a half-and-half mix with lavender or chamomile for its antifungal, anti-inflammatory, and antiseptic capabilities.

Chamomile flower Antifungal, soothing, and cleansing, chamomile flower is the best way to reduce frequent inflammation. The infusion is especially recommended for the fragile skin around the eyes.

Elder flower A gentle cleanser, toner, and astringent, elder flower may also be used to reduce inflammation.

Lavender flower Though slightly drying, lavender soothes, reduces inflammation, and cleanses.

Lime (or linden) flower Similar to chamomile, lime flower is very calming. Its mildly toning, anti-inflammatory effect is beneficial for aging skin.

Mallow Its gentle anti-inflammatory properties make mallow a wonderful way to soothe and calm irritated skin.

Mint Use this herb to tone the skin.

Rosemary Antiseptic, toning, and vitalizing, rosemary improves blood circulation in the capillaries. Use alone or in a half-and-half mix with yarrow for a more astringent effect.

Thyme A strong anti-bacterial herb, thyme is effective as a skin wash for acne or infected eczema. Use alone or in equal parts with chamomile and/or calendula to soothe and heal.

Yarrow Particularly good for aging or damaged skin, yarrow is recognized as a toner, astringent, and antiseptic.

TO MAKE A SIMPLE INFUSION
Use one generous tablespoon of dried chopped herbs to 9fl.oz. (250ml)

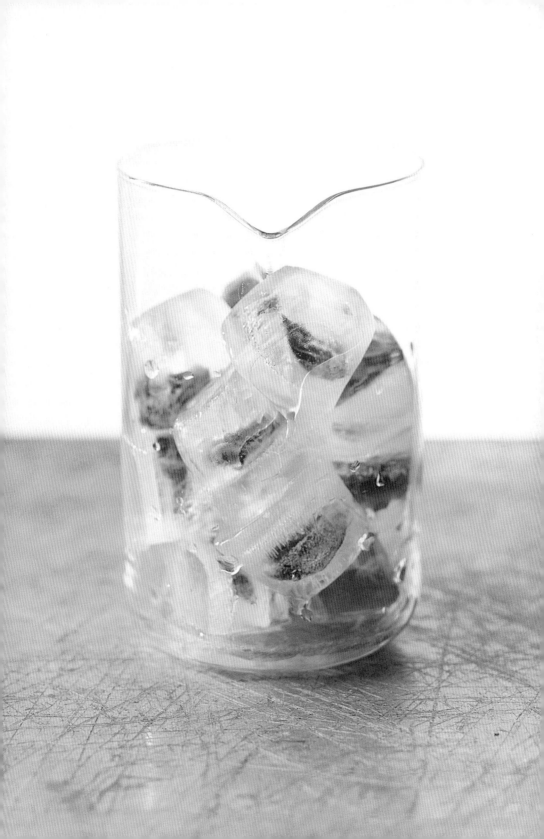

of boiling water. Place the herbs in a mug and fill it to the brim with the water. Infuse for 10 minutes, strain, reserve the liquid, and allow to cool before using. Apply with cotton pads or in a mister and leave to dry naturally.

INFUSIONS FOR ICE CUBES

An infusion has a shelf life of about 12 hours, so don't be tempted to bottle large quantities. However, you can freeze a strained and cooled infusion in an ice-cube tray and keep it in the freezer compartment of your refrigerator for up to 1 month or in the freezer for up to 3 months. The recommended infusions for ice cubes are chamomile, lavender, lime flower, and rosemary. The hydrosols listed on page 45 can also be diluted to make ice cubes. Allow 1 tablespoon of hydrosol per 3½fl.oz (100ml) of bottled or spring water.

To use, simply rub a cube directly on your face, neck, and arms for a deliciously cooling and hydrating effect. This also has a toning action because it quickens blood circulation in the capillaries of the dermis.

INFUSIONS FOR COMPRESSES

Compresses tone the skin—improving blood circulation, hydrating, and closing the pores—and calm inflammation. Especially good for dry, aging, or damaged skin, they can be used occasionally on any skin type.

Ideally, you need two large bowls, but you may be able to improvise with one bowl and a bathroom basin. You also need two small face towels. Place 1 generous tablespoon of any of the dried herbs listed on page 30 and 1 tablespoon of lemon juice in one of the bowls, and cover with 3 cups of boiling water. Infuse for 15 minutes. Into the second bowl pour about 2 pints (1 liter) of cold water and 1 tablespoon of apple cider vinegar. Add a few ice cubes to chill.

Immerse one of the towels in the hot infusion and squeeze out the excess water before laying the towel on the face and leaving it for about 1 minute. Take care: It will be hot at first. Remove the first towel and quickly dip the other towel into the cold water bowl. Apply to the face in the same way, again leaving for 1 minute. Repeat this procedure twice, alternating hot and cold compresses. It is important to finish with a cold compress to close the pores. Finish by dabbing on rose hydrosol (see page 45) and allowing to dry naturally.

steaming

One traditional and very simple way to deep clean the skin is to steam your face for a few minutes from time to time. Steaming removes dirt and pollution very efficiently from the skin, but it removes important natural oils as well. So, although the technique brings excellent results on an oily skin or for anyone suffering from acne, most skin types must bear in mind that in the long term it has a drying effect.

Steaming should not be used too often on dry or aging skin (once a month is the maximum) and never for more than 2 to 3 minutes. On oily skin, it can be done once or twice every seven days, and for 6 to 8 minutes at a time. For combination skin, 2 to 3 minutes once a week is the recommended maximum. Normal skin will benefit from an occasional steaming (every two weeks), as long as the exposure to steam is not prolonged (5 minutes maximum). It is not recommended for extremely sensitive skin; for anyone suffering from severe inflammation, infection, sunburn, or rosacea; or for those who have many small blood vessels visible on the surface of the skin. However, these conditions respond very well to the regular application of clay masks (see the cleansing recipes for dry or aging skin).

TO STEAM

All you need is a large bowl containing about 2 pints (1 liter) of boiling water and a medium-sized towel. Sit before the bowl, cover your head with the towel, and keep your face in the steam for the recommended time. Then, pat your face dry with cotton pads or a towel and tone with rose hydrosol (see page 45), allowing the skin to dry naturally.

The benefits of steaming can be enhanced by adding two drops of chamomile, geranium, lavender, rose otto, or tea tree essential oil (see pages 34 and 40–41) to the boiling water. After drying, apply a thin film of the same oil to the skin, diluted in a calendula carrier (see pages 34–37).

aromatherapy

Essential oils are an excellent and safe alternative to cosmetic and conventional medical treatment of the skin. They have been used for years with great success to treat the most difficult cases of eczema and rosacea, but they are also irreplaceable for daily skin care. For confirmation, you only have to look at the ingredient list on most cosmetic products. In this book, you will find essential and carrier oils used in the recipe sections—to cleanse, nourish, and tone; for steaming (see page 33); for massage (see page 42–44); and for the treatment of common skin conditions (see pages 114–125).

ESSENTIAL OILS

Found in the roots, leaves, stems, or flowers of aromatic plants; in the bark of trees, such as pine, fir, and cinnamon; and in the peel of some citrus fruits, essential oils are a complex mixture of up to 250 chemicals. These fragrant substances, synthesized in plants by the energy of the sun, are usually extracted by the ancient process of steam distillation. A few (for example, the citrus oils) are obtained by cold expression; rose absolute is derived by chemical extraction and is inferior to the recommended form, rose otto.

They have such a complex chemistry that it remains impossible to know exactly how they work. But, scientific analysis in the late twentieth century classified the families of molecules commonly found in essential oils, and that has helped to explain some of the therapeutic effects consistently observed in aromatherapy, such as the destruction or inhibition of viruses and bacteria, anti-inflammatory action, and hormone regulation.

CARRIER OILS

Because of their powerful effects, essential oils are only very rarely used undiluted directly on the skin (see "safety precautions" on page 36). Much gentler vegetable oils are used to dilute the essential oils used for massage. These are known as carrier oils. Although any vegetable oil could be used, cold-pressed oils obtained from nuts or seeds are preferred for their therapeutic properties and because they can act in synergy with specific essential oils for additional benefits. Cold-pressed oils are expensive, but they are much more beneficial than the cheaper, industrially extracted oils, containing varying but larger quantities of valuable vitamins, trace elements, and fatty acids. They are also economical in use—a little bit goes a long way.

CHOOSING CARRIER OILS

The first step in choosing oils for massage or to treat common skin problems is to select a carrier (or carriers). A chart listing the characteristics of all the major carrier oils appears on pages 38–39. The programs in "Caring for your skin" give the appropriate carrier oils for each skin type and every age group (see pages 14–19). Sweet almond and olive oil will suit any kind of skin and can serve either as a single carrier or as the larger part of a blend of carriers.

It is very important to choose the right carrier oil: Though carrier oils have a specific action, they can also diffuse or enhance the therapeutic qualities of the essential oils they carry. When selecting a carrier oil for massage, try one oil at a time. If it feels right, it probably is—so long as you've assessed your skin type and its condition correctly (see page 12). You may sometimes need to blend two, possibly three, carriers that suit your skin type, age group, and skin condition, but most of the time only one is needed. Blends of two or three carrier oils are used for their therapeutic effects, or for economy.

Therapeutically, for example, calendula oil works well in synergy with hypericum oil for very oily, damaged, or inflamed skin. And for reasons of economy, blends are usually no more than 10 to 15 percent jojoba or macadamia nut carrier oils, or borage, evening primrose, rosehip seed, or vitamin E supplementary oils, combined with a cheaper carrier such as apricot kernel, olive, or sweet almond oil.

Quality olive, sweet almond, and wheat germ oils are easily available, while the others can be ordered from reputable specialty shops (see page 126).

CHOOSING ESSENTIAL OILS

You can use a blend of up to four essential oils in the single or blended carrier oils used for massage, or to treat common skin conditions. A chart listing all the essential oils recommended and their main benefits appears on pages 40–41. The programs for lifelong skin care in "Caring for your skin" give the appropriate essential oils for each skin type and age group (see pages 14–19).

The principal oil for any blend of essential oils for massage must satisfy your main objective: for example, to hydrate the skin, or to regulate excessive sebum. You may then choose smaller amounts of one or two other oils that will enhance and complement the action of your principal oil. Finally, one more oil can be selected either as a balancer—to counteract any possible over-action of the other oils—or to treat some other symptom of your skin. The selected essential oils are measured and blended in a separate container before being added in the required quantity to your carrier: The total amount of essential oil should never be more than 3.5 percent of the resulting preparation. See opposite for detailed instructions on blending oils.

SAFETY PRECAUTIONS

Most essential oils are safe for home use if they are used correctly. However, experts have conflicting opinions on the uses of essential oils by pregnant and nursing women. Essential oils may stimulate the uterus. A woman who is pregnant or nursing should avoid all essential oils unless otherwise directed by her health care practitioner. Essential oils are intended for external use only. Essential oils are concentrated substances, so keep them out of children's reach. Never leave a bottle without a secure dropper where a child could drink the contents. Avoid contact with wood furniture.

Unless personally advised by an expert, and with the few following exceptions, never apply undiluted essential oil to the skin. It must be diluted in a carrier oil first. But lavender can be used undiluted on burns; tea tree, on athlete's foot; and rose otto or sandalwood, as a perfume.

Avoid immediate exposure to strong sunlight or ultraviolet light after using citrus oils, such as mandarin. They are slightly phototoxic, which means they can cause skin discoloration, so use them with caution. Juniper should always be used sparingly as it can sometimes cause mild skin irritation.

Most essential oils, even when diluted, will cause stinging if they get into the eyes. If you splash undiluted essential oil into your eyes, flush them immediately with milk or with a carrier or vegetable oil and, if the stinging and irritation continues, seek medical assistance quickly. If the essential oil is diluted, flush immediately with a carrier oil.

BLENDING OILS

While you are experimenting with various mixes, it is best to make enough for just one day's massage. Two teaspoons (10ml) of carrier oil and ten drops of essential oil are all you need. Consult the recommendations for your skin type and age on pages 14–19 and the charts on pages 38–41 to select the appropriate carrier and essential oils. To keep it simple at first, choose a single carrier and two essential oils (5 drops of each).

Once you are satisfied with a particular blend, it makes sense to prepare a larger amount—these oils have a shelf life of about three months. For the contents of a 2-tablespoon (30ml) bottle of carrier oil(s), you will need an essential oil blend totaling 10 drops; for a 3½-tablespoon (50ml) bottle of carrier oil(s), the essential oils will total 15 drops. (Viscosities vary but on average 1ml = 20 drops of essential oil.)

To blend oils in quantity, you need two colored glass bottles—light degrades the benefits of essential oils. You will find them in aromatherapy shops and many local pharmacies (see page 126 for mail-order suppliers). One must be large enough to hold your assembled preparation, but the other can be very small. This one will be used to blend your essential oils before they are added to the carrier(s), and it needs a removable dropper as well as a top.

Begin by pouring the required amount of carrier oil(s) into the large bottle. Then combine the essential oils in the small bottle, close (using the dropper/top), and shake well. Finally, add the essential oils to the carrier bottle, close, and shake again to blend. Your oil mix is now ready to use.

carrier oils

••••• = very useful
• = slightly useful
o = not useful

	for normal skin	for dry skin	for oily skin	for combination skin	for aging skin	for sensitive skin
apricot kernel	•••	•••••	•	••••	•••••	•••
* calendula	•••	•	•••••	•••	••	•••••
hazelnut	••••	••	••••	••••	•••	•••
* hypericum (St. John's Wort)	•••	••	••••	•••	•••	••••
jojoba	•	•••	•••	•••	•	•••
lime (or linden) blossom	••	•••	•	•••	•••••	•••••
macadamia nut	•	•••	••••	•••	•••	••
olive	•••••	•••••	•••••	•••••	•••••	••••
sweet almond	•••••	••••	•••	•••••	••••	••••
wheat germ	••	••••	•	•••	•••••	••••
borage or evening primrose	••	•••	•	•	•••••	•••••
rosehip seed	••	•••••	o	••	•••••	•••••
vitamin e	••	•••••	•	••	•••••	••••

* Infuse in the carrier oil of your choice

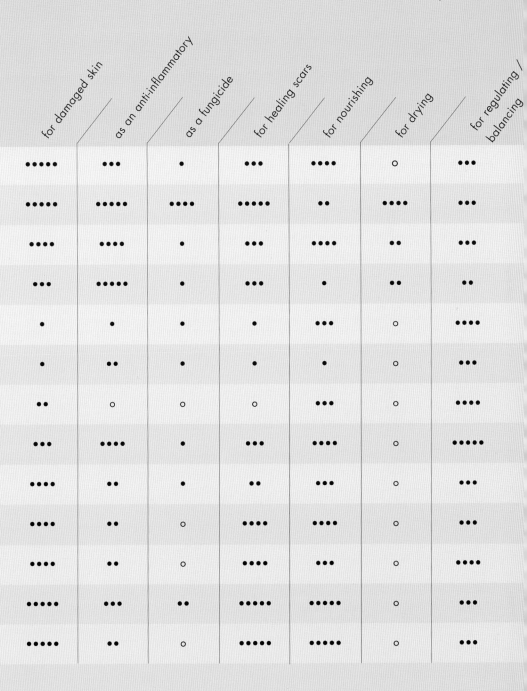

This table and that on pages 40–41 represent a broad evaluation based on practical experience.
Supplementary oils are listed in italic and can be added in small quantities to carrier oils (see page 35).

essential oils

••••• = very useful
• = slightly useful
o = not useful

	for normal skin	for dry skin	for oily skin	for combination skin	for aging skin	for sensitive skin	for damaged skin	as an anti-inflammatory
cedarwood	••	•	••	••	••	o	•••••	o
*chamomile german	••	•	•••	•••	•••	•••••	•••••	•••••
*chamomile roman	••	•	•••	•••	•••	•••••	•••	•••
clary sage	••	•••	••	••	•••••	•••	•••	•
cypress	••	•	•••••	••	••••	••	•••	o
frankincense	••	••••	••	••	••••	••	•••••	•••
geranium	•••	•••••	•••	•	••••	•••	•••	•••
juniper	•	•	•••	••	•	o	••	•
lavender	•••	••	•••••	••••	•••	••••	•••••	••••
lemon	••	••	••••	•••	••••	•	••••	••
mandarin	••	•	•••••	•••	•••	••••	••	•
myrrh	••	•••••	•••	•••	•••	•	••••	•••
neroli	•••	••••	•	••	••••	•••	•••	••
niaouli	•••	•••	•••	•••	•••	•	••	•••
palmarosa	•••	•••	••	•••	•••	••	•••	••••
patchouli	••	•••	•••	•••	•••	o	•••	•••
rosemary	•••	•••	•••	•••	••••	••	•••••	•••
rose otto	•••	•••	••	•••	•••••	•••	•••	•••
rosewood	•••	•••	•••	•••		••••	•••	••
sandalwood	•••	•••	••	•••	••	•••	••	•
tea tree	•••	••	•••	•••	••	•••	•••	•••

*Use either where chamomile is specified. German chamomile is more concentrated.

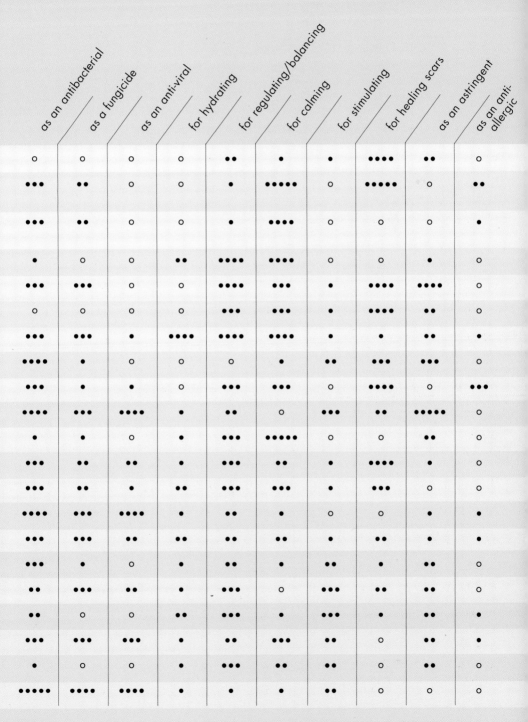

NOTE: Pregnant and nursing women should avoid essential oils unless otherwise directed by a health care practitioner.

MASSAGE TECHNIQUE

Regular massage with an appropriate blend of carrier and essential oils is an essential part of any good skin maintenance program. An effective way to tone and generally improve the condition of any type of skin, it works by relaxing all the small muscles of the face, improving the circulation, breaking down fatty deposits in the lower levels of the skin, and releasing toxins. Remember to make good use of massage in association with masks and lotions as recommended for your skin type or condition (see pages 14–19 and 114–125). The sequence that follows repeats several simple techniques.

Technique 1 Use the tips of the index, middle, and ring fingers together to exert·a deep, local pressure in a tiny circular movement. You should be able to feel the skin rubbing against the small muscles of the face. Lift the fingers and reposition them to travel across the skin.

Technique 2 Use the flat pads of the index, middle, and ring fingers together or simply the thumb to travel across the skin—either in a slow, spiraling action or by simply sliding upward, downward or outward. For the most part, keep the remainder of your hand resting lightly on the face.

Pinching Use your index finger and thumb lightly but with enough strength to stimulate the circulation and cause a slight change of skin color. Beware of bruising—pinch lightly on the eyebrows and upper face, more heavily along the jaw.

FACIAL MASSAGE SEQUENCE

Make sure you are sitting comfortably with everything you need at hand: a headband or combs to secure your hair away from your face, a wet, soft cloth to dampen your skin so that the oils emulsify and penetrate more easily, and a little massage oil poured onto a plate.

Warm-up Starting on either side of the nose, pinch along each eyebrow and as far as possible along the temples toward the tops of the ears. Then pinch from the chin, working slowly along the jaw line and up to the base of the ears. Do this three times.

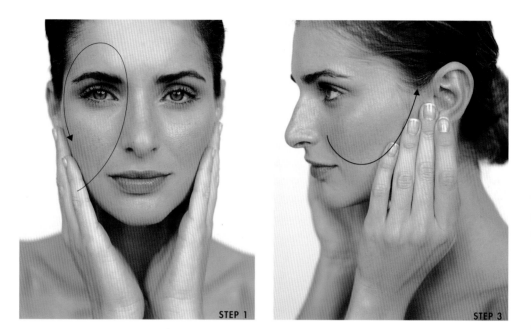

STEP 1

STEP 3

Dip the pads of your fingers into the oil, and rub your palms together to spread it evenly. Place your fingertips on your jawbone and with light pressure, make a large, sweeping circle from the jaw line up either side of the nose to the center of the forehead, out along the hairline, and then down the temples to meet at the jawbone. This gently stimulates energy and spreads the oil.

With the tips of all three fingers and the local pressure of Technique 1, start at the chin and travel along the jaw line and then up from the angles of the jaw to the temples. Do this three times.

Using the pads of the three fingers and the small spiraling movement of Technique 2, begin on each side of the nose, close to the base of the nostrils, moving first under the cheekbones and then up toward the tops of the ears.

Placing the tips of the middle fingers at the inner corners of the eyes, slide your fingers upward, pushing against the orbital bone, and then outward, just above the eyebrows, towards the ears.

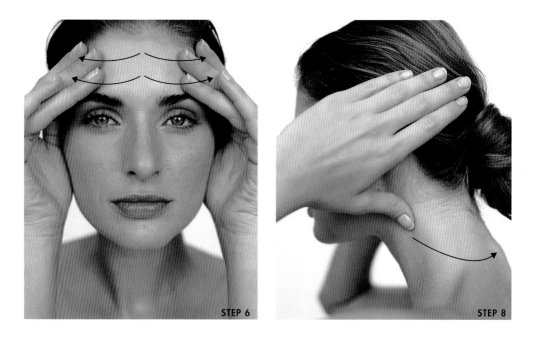

STEP 6

STEP 8

5   Use the pads of all three fingers and the spiraling movement of
Technique 2 to massage the forehead, starting just above the top
of the nose, moving up toward the hairline, and then outward along it
until you reach the temples.

6   Using Technique 2, position the pads of all three fingers at the
base of the central frown line, just above the top of the nose, and
slide them toward the temples. Do this three times.

7   Massage your scalp firmly, as if you were shampooing your hair.
Begin at the temples and work downward, behind the ears and
towards the base of the skull.

8   Resting your palms on your ears so that the thumbs point
downward, massage from your throat to the nape of the neck in a
broad, spiraling version of Technique 2. Do this three times.

9   Place one hand, palm down, on each side of your nose. Your
fingertips should rest slightly above your eyebrows. With firm, even
pressure, slide your hands outward toward the ears. Do this three times.

10   Bring the sequence to an end by repeating the sweeping
movement described in step 1.

hydrosols

Also known as floral waters (but *not* flower waters), hydrosols are a by-product of steam distillation, created while extracting essential oil. Hydrosols have properties similar to those of their related essential oils, although inevitably in a less concentrated form, but they are enriched with various water-soluble active ingredients. Their gentleness makes them an excellent way to tone, hydrate, and rebalance the pH of the skin, so they are frequently recommended as final cleansers/toners after cleansing or nourishing masks. Most also have a bactericidal and antiviral action and can disinfect sensitive or damaged skin without the harshness of detergents or alcohol-based lotions. All are available from specialty shops or by mail order (see page 126).

USING HYDROSOLS

Hydrosols can be applied to the face twice daily. Use cotton pads or or a mister, but be careful to avoid the eyes. Allow to dry naturally. Hydrosols can also be added to a bath as a general skin tonic (use 3 tablespoons) and are sometimes substituted for water in preparing clay masks (see page 23).

Chamomile Suitable for all skin types, chamomile is a very gentle anti-inflammatory, good for over-exposure to sun and wind.

Clary sage Suitable for dry and aging skin, clary sage relieves skin problems associated with fluctuating hormone levels and menopause.

Cornflower See chamomile. Cornflower is often used around the eyes because, unlike most hydrosols, it does not burn in contact with them.

Lavender Though slightly drying, lavender is suitable for all skin types. It has cooling, anti-inflammatory properties that can ease sun- or wind-burn.

Orange blossom (neroli) Inflammation-reducing, this hydrosol is particularly good at soothing dry or sensitive skin and for treating rosacea.

Rose Appropriate for all skin types, especially aging, rose is recognized for its balancing, tonic, and astringent properties.

Rosemary Excellent for balancing and toning all skin types, rosemary stimulates circulation and is a superb hydrosol for hair.

Witch hazel Suitable for all skin types, witch hazel is mildly astringent.

apple cider vinegar

The use of vinegar with a variety of plants or essential oils for cosmetic purposes can be traced back to the Romans and was fashionable during the nineteenth century as *vinaigre de toilette*.

Vinegar has a tonic action that promotes blood circulation in the small capillaries that irrigate the skin. It is also antiseptic, preventing the proliferation of bacteria, viruses, or yeast that trigger infection. It can dissolve excessive fatty deposits at the surface of the skin and reduce scaly or peeling conditions. Lastly, vinegar regulates the pH of the skin. Vinegar is most effective when used with lavender, rosemary, rose, or elder flower. It is essential to use top-quality white wine or cider vinegar. Dry any fresh plant material for two days before using.

Measure and mix any dried plant material and then add the vinegar and any blended essential oils (see pages 34 and 37). Apple ciders composed entirely of liquids can be used at once. Those containing plant material must be left to macerate. Prepare the latter in a screwtop jar and leave on a window sill as instructed, strain, and then bottle. To use, add 1 teaspoon of apple cider to a cup of bottled or spring water to wash your face or pour 3–4 tablespoons into a bath.

LAVENDER, ROSEMARY AND ROSEWOOD

VINEGAR	17½fl.oz (500ml) good-quality white wine or apple cider vinegar
ESSENTIAL OILS	⅗ teaspoon each lavender and rosemary, ⅖ teaspoon rosewood
PLUS	2 tablespoons glycerin

CALENDULA AND ELDER FLOWER

PLANT MATERIAL	2oz (50g) calendula flowers and 3oz (75g) elder flowers
VINEGAR	2 pints (1 liter) good-quality white wine or apple cider vinegar
MACERATE	2 weeks

LAVENDER, ROSE, PINK, AND LIME

PLANT MATERIAL	1oz (30g) each lavender and lime (or linden) flowers, rose petals, pinks
VINEGAR	2 pints (1 liter) good-quality white wine or apple cider vinegar
MACERATE	2 weeks

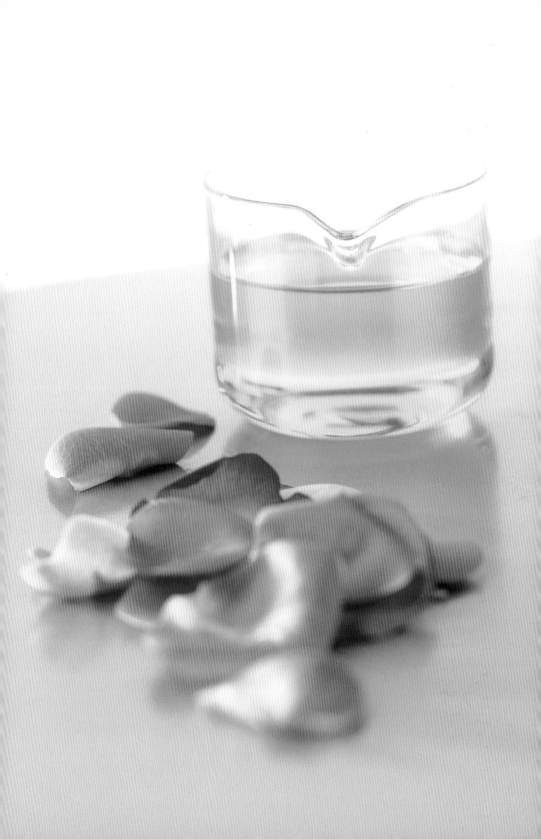

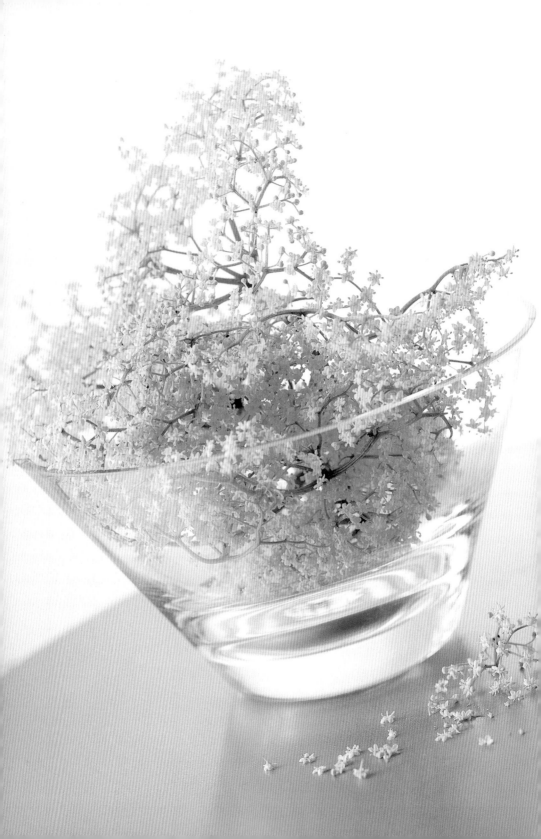

cleansing
recipes

traditional almond milk

The use of almond milk for the skin can be traced back to the Egyptian pharaohs. As beneficial today as it was then, this gentle lotion nourishes as it cleanses. Almonds contain a variety of trace elements, vitamins A and B, and oleic and linoleic acids (or vitamin F), two of the polyunsaturated fatty acids that are vital for healthy skin. Honey boosts the nourishing effect with additional trace elements and enzymes. Throw away any left over after a week.

INGREDIENTS
2oz (50g) ground almonds
2 tablespoons organic honey
17½fl.oz (500ml) bottled or spring water

METHOD
Add the ground almonds and honey to the bottled or spring water and stir well until the honey has dissolved. Set aside for 2 hours. Filter, pour into a covered container or bottle, and store in a refrigerator.

Apply generously to the face and neck, using a cotton pad, and leave on for 20 minutes—time for the lotion to penetrate the skin and dry naturally.

EFFECT	cleanses, nourishes
SKIN TYPES	all, especially dry and aging
FREQUENCY OF USE	twice daily
SHELF LIFE	1 week in refrigerator
PREPARATION TIME	10 minutes, plus 2 hours "resting time"
TREATMENT TIME	20 minutes

clay and witch hazel eye mask

This astringent mask is particularly useful for the fragile skin around the eyes. To use on the face and neck, multiply all the quantities by three, and see page 29 for application and removal. For hydrosols, see page 45; for clay, see pages 22–24.

INGREDIENTS
1 tablespoon witch hazel hydrosol
1 tablespoon cornflower hydrosol
1 tablespoon white or green clay powder
bottled or spring water

METHOD
Following the basic method described on page 23, add the witch hazel and cornflower hydrosols to the clay and set aside for 30 minutes without stirring. Then mix well to make a smooth paste.

Apply a thin layer very gently around the eyes and leave on for 10 minutes. Rinse carefully with bottled or spring water and pat dry.

VARIATION
Substitute rose hydrosol for the cornflower for a more toning effect. To moisturize, dab apricot oil or rosehip seed oil around the eyes as an aftercare treatment.

EFFECT	cleanses, tones, reduces inflammation
SKIN TYPES	all
FREQUENCY OF USE	twice daily for 2 weeks
SHELF LIFE	8 hours in refrigerator
PREPARATION TIME	10 minutes, plus 30 minutes "resting time"
TREATMENT TIME	eyes: 10 minutes; face and neck: 20 minutes

fresh orange juice and clay mask

Orange is the gentlest of the astringent citrus juices. Rich in vitamins B and C, calcium, potassium, phosphorus, manganese, copper, zinc, and antioxidants, it is an excellent substitute for water in a clay mask. For clay, see pages 22–24; for hydrosols, see page 45.

INGREDIENTS
1 medium orange
2 tablespoons white or green clay powder
bottled or spring water
witch hazel hydrosol

METHOD
Slice and press the orange to extract 3 tablespoons of juice. Following the standard method described on page 23, add the orange juice to the clay and set aside for 30 minutes before stirring. Then mix thoroughly for a smooth paste.

For application to the face and neck, see page 29. After 20 minutes, rinse off, using bottled or spring water and cotton pads, and pat dry. Dab on witch hazel and allow to dry naturally.

VARIATION
Use grapefruit juice for a more astringent, light bleaching action on freckles or the brown spots of aging skin.

EFFECT	cleanses, tones
SKIN TYPES	all
FREQUENCY OF USE	daily
SHELF LIFE	6 hours in refrigerator
PREPARATION TIME	10 minutes, plus 30 minutes "resting time"
TREATMENT TIME	20 minutes

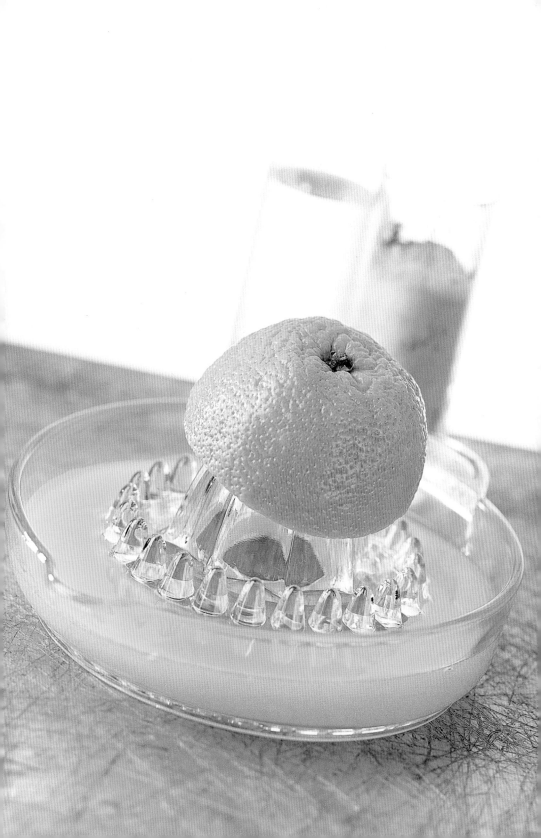

honey and cucumber cleansing milk

This simple recipe cleans the skin while reducing inflammation. The milk contains lactic acid, an excellent natural cleanser with a revitalizing, balancing effect on the pH of the skin. The honey is rich in nourishing trace elements, and the cucumber juice hydrates and reduces inflammation. For infusions, see page 30.

INGREDIENTS

¼ small cucumber
2 tablespoons organic honey
1 tablespoon fresh whole milk
bottled or spring water or chamomile infusion

METHOD

Peel and seed the cucumber. Purée the flesh, using a food processor or blender, and extract 2 tablespoons of juice by straining through a piece of muslin. Stir the honey into the juice. Once they are well mixed, add the milk and stir again.

Apply the lotion evenly to the face and neck, using cotton pads. Leave on for 20 minutes before rinsing off with bottled or spring water or a chamomile infusion and cotton pads. Pat dry.

EFFECT	cleanses, reduces inflammation, nourishes, hydrates
SKIN TYPES	all
FREQUENCY OF USE	once or twice daily
SHELF LIFE	6 hours in refrigerator
PREPARATION TIME	5 minutes
TREATMENT TIME	20 minutes

clay and cucumber cleansing mask

A fast-acting cooler for inflamed skin, this recipe is especially useful for eczema and rosacea. The astringent grapefruit juice is both bleaching and toning. For clay, see pages 22–24; for hydrosols, see page 45; for infusions, see page 30; for carrier oils, see pages 34 and 38.

INGREDIENTS

½ **medium cucumber**

½ **grapefruit**

2 tablespoons white or green clay powder

bottled or spring water

rose hydrosol or chamomile infusion

METHOD

Peel and purée the cucumber in a food processor or blender and then strain through a piece of muslin, reserving 2 tablespoons of juice. Extract 1 tablespoon of juice from the half grapefruit. Following the clay mask method described on page 23, substitute the cucumber juice and grapefuit juice for the water and set aside for 30 minutes without stirring. Mix to a smooth paste.

For application to the face and neck and removal, see page 29; rinse off with bottled or spring water. Finish with rosewater hydrosol or an infusion of chamomile and allow to dry naturally.

VARIATION

For dry skin, omit the grapefruit juice and stir 1 tablespoon of sweet almond oil into the smooth paste.

EFFECT	cleanses, reduces inflammation, tones
SKIN TYPES	all (see VARIATION for dry skin)
FREQUENCY OF USE	once or twice a week
SHELF LIFE	8 hours in refrigerator
PREPARATION TIME	10 minutes, plus 30 minutes "resting time"
TREATMENT TIME	20 minutes

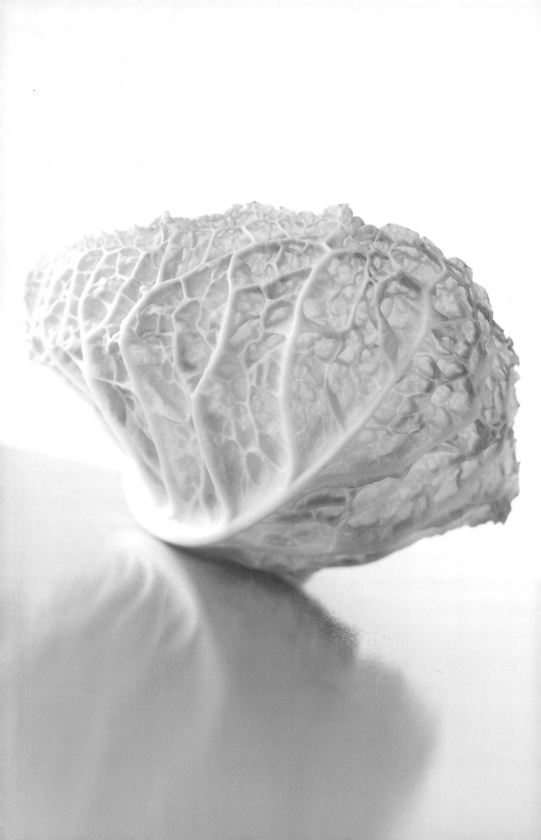

fresh cabbage leaf cleanser

The virtues of the cabbage—rich in vitamins A, B, C, E, and K; potassium; sulphur; and copper—have been known for thousands of years. Its vegetable acids and minerals have a deeply cleansing effect. This mask is particularly good for acne, eczema, or overexposure to wind or sun. For carrier oils, see pages 34 and 38; for hydrosols, see page 45.

INGREDIENTS

¼ **small green cabbage**

2 tablespoons fresh carrot juice

½ **lemon**

1 tablespoon olive oil

2 tablespoons white or green clay powder

bottled or spring water

rose hydrosol

METHOD

Discard the outer leaves of the cabbage. Chop the remainder, rinse, and pat dry. If making your own carrot juice, prepare 2 tablespoons. Press the lemon to extract 1 teaspoon of juice. Combine the cabbage, carrot juice, lemon, and olive oil in a blender or food processor and blend to a smooth purée. Add 3 tablespoons of the purée to the clay and stir to mix.

Apply to the face and neck and leave on for 20 minutes. Rinse with bottled or spring water and cotton pads and pat dry. Dab on a little rose hydrosol, and allow to dry naturally.

EFFECT	cleanses, heals, reduces inflammation
SKIN TYPES	all
FREQUENCY OF USE	once a week, or daily for inflamed or damaged skin
SHELF LIFE	24 hours in refrigerator
PREPARATION TIME	10 minutes
TREATMENT TIME	20 minutes

white or green clay cleansing milk

This cleanser has a very slight drying action, which makes it particularly suitable for use on oily or combination skin. For clay, see pages 22–24; for infusions, see page 30.

INGREDIENTS

1 tablespoon white or green clay powder
9fl.oz (250ml) bottled or spring water

METHOD

Simply add the clay to the bottled or spring water and store in a covered container or bottle in the refrigerator.

Shake before use and apply evenly to the face, neck, and hands, using cotton pads. Leave on for 20 minutes to penetrate the skin and allow to dry naturally.

VARIATION

For an anti-inflammatory effect, use a chamomile infusion instead of bottled or spring water.

EFFECT	cleanses
SKIN TYPES	normal, oily, combination
FREQUENCY OF USE	twice daily
SHELF LIFE	1 week in refrigerator
PREPARATION TIME	5 minutes
TREATMENT TIME	20 minutes

rose hydrosol and lemon juice cleanser

Lemon juice is a very effective cleanser and toner. The most powerful astringent of the citric fruit acids, it also contains vitamin B_3 (a strong astringent), which inhibits bacterial action on the skin. In this recipe, lemon toughens up rose hydrosol's gentler balancing and tonic action. Good-quality hydrosol is essential; it is now widely available from specialty shops and by mail order (see page 126). For more about hydrosols, see page 45.

INGREDIENTS
½ **lemon**
3½fl.oz (100ml) rose hydrosol

METHOD
Press the lemon to extract 1 teaspoon of juice and simply add the juice to the rose hydrosol. Store in a covered container or bottle in the refrigerator.

Apply twice a day to the face and neck, using cotton pads. Transfer to a spray bottle if you prefer to mist the skin. Leave on to penetrate and allow to dry naturally.

EFFECT	cleanses, tones
SKIN TYPES	oily, combination
FREQUENCY OF USE	twice daily
SHELF LIFE	1 week in refrigerator
PREPARATION TIME	2 minutes
TREATMENT TIME	20 minutes

fresh milk and tomato juice cleanser

Good tomatoes are an abundant source of vitamins A, B (including folic acid), and C; potassium and magnesium; and valuable antioxidants and trace elements. The high acid content in the recipe—lactic acid in the milk and fruit acid in the tomato—gives this cleansing lotion a gentle peeling action. Test on the inside arm or wrist for any possible allergic reactions before using on the face. For infusions, see page 30.

INGREDIENTS
1 medium very ripe tomato
5fl.oz (150ml) fresh whole milk
bottled or spring water or chamomile infusion

METHOD
Process the tomato, using a food processor or blender. Strain through a piece of muslin and discard the pulp. Add the tomato juice to an equal amount of milk. Store in a covered container or bottle in the refrigerator.

Apply to the face and neck, using cotton pads, once or twice a day. Leave on for 10 minutes and rinse with bottled or spring water or an infusion of chamomile and pat dry.

EFFECT	cleanses
SKIN TYPES	oily, combination (but test first, see above)
	not recommended for sensitive skin
FREQUENCY OF USE	once or twice daily for 1 week
SHELF LIFE	6 hours in refrigerator
PREPARATION TIME	5 minutes
TREATMENT TIME	10 minutes

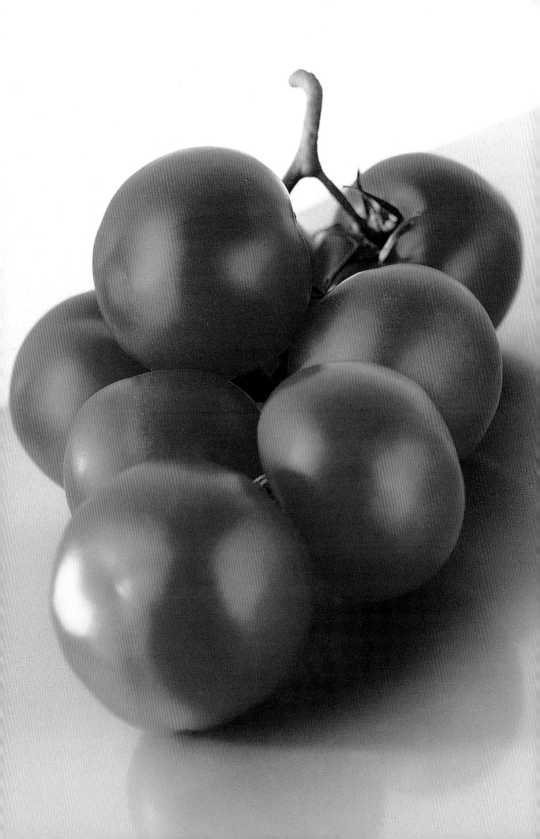

rose hydrosol and witch hazel cleanser

A traditional cleansing recipe, this one also has a strong toning action. Applied lightly around the eyes, it helps to reduce the faint lines of expression that begin to appear in the mid-20s. But be careful— hydrosols contain distilled essential oils, and even in this form they can make your eyes sting if applied carelessly. The cleanser can also be used as a general toner on aging skin. For hydrosols, see page 45.

INGREDIENTS
7fl.oz (200ml) rose hydrosol
3½fl.oz (100ml) witch hazel hydrosol

METHOD
Measure the hydrosols into a bottle, close tightly, and shake well to mix. This preparation can be kept for several weeks, and there's no need to store it in a refrigerator.

Apply carefully twice a day, using cotton pads. Leave on for 20 minutes and allow to dry naturally.

EFFECT	cleanses, tones, reduces inflammation
SKIN TYPES	all (see above)
FREQUENCY OF USE	twice daily
SHELF LIFE	1 month
PREPARATION TIME	2 minutes
TREATMENT TIME	20 minutes

elder and orange blossom cleanser

Orange blossom, also known as neroli, is particularly good for dry skin, and elder flower is good for aging or inflamed skin. Here they combine with apple cider vinegar's regulating effect on the pH of the skin and its tonic action on the tiny blood vessels that serve the dermis in a recipe that vitalizes as it cleanses. For more about vinegar, see page 46; for hydrosols, see page 45.

INGREDIENTS

1 tablespoon dried elder flowers
3½ tablespoons apple cider vinegar
5fl.oz (150ml) orange blossom hydrosol

METHOD

Place the elder flowers in a small bowl and cover with apple cider vinegar. Soak for 1 hour. Discard the flowers and add the apple cider vinegar to the orange blossom hydrosol. Store in a closed brown glass bottle.

Apply to the face and neck, using cotton pads, and allow to dry naturally.

EFFECT	cleanses, tones, balances pH
SKIN TYPES	all
FREQUENCY OF USE	once or twice daily
SHELF LIFE	1 month
PREPARATION TIME	5 minutes, plus 1 hour soaking time
TREATMENT TIME	10 minutes

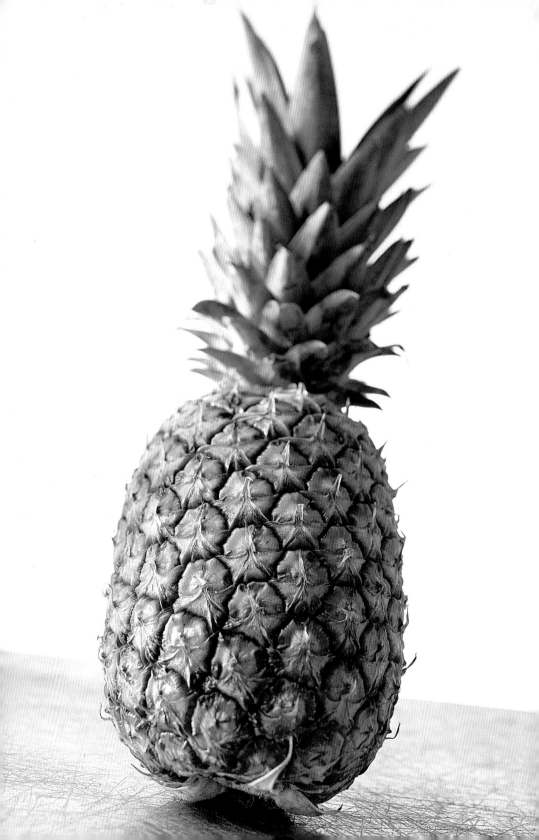

pineapple exfoliating mask

An excellent way to use the tougher, sometimes inedible, central section of the pineapple, this mask acts as a gentle peeling agent.
Pineapple is rich in vitamins A, B (including folic acid), and C; potassium, magnesium, manganese, iron, and sulphur; plus a particularly
effective combination of citric and malic fruit acids and enzymes.
Although it may irritate sensitive skin slightly, allergic reactions to
pineapple are rare, and the chamomile infusion and anti-inflammatory
oatmeal will counteract the effect. For infusions, see page 30.

INGREDIENTS

1 ripe medium pineapple
1 cup chamomile infusion, cooled
2–3 tablespoons oatmeal flakes
bottled or spring water

METHOD

Peel the pineapple and cut it in half lengthwise. Remove the pithy
central section, using a knife or spoon, and purée it in a food processor
or blender. Stir 2 tablespoons of chamomile infusion into the purée,
mixing well, and then stir in enough oatmeal flakes to make a smooth
paste.

Apply to the face and neck, avoiding the area around the eyes,
and leave on for 15 minutes. Rinse with bottled or spring water, using
cotton pads. Dab on some of the remaining chamomile infusion and
allow to dry naturally.

EFFECT	cleanses
SKIN TYPES	all (see above for sensitive skin)
FREQUENCY OF USE	once a week
SHELF LIFE	12 hours in refrigerator
PREPARATION TIME	5 minutes
TREATMENT TIME	15 minutes

strawberry and almond oil cleanser

Use this recipe to remove makeup, cleanse, and tone. The fruit acid in the strawberries acts as a gentle peeling agent and astringent, while the sweet almond oil counterbalances the effect, preventing too aggressive an action. If you have sensitive skin, test the lotion on the inside arm or wrist. For carrier oils, see pages 34 and 38; for infusions, see page 30.

INGREDIENTS

6 large, very ripe strawberries

2 tablespoons sweet almond oil

bottled or spring water or chamomile infusion

METHOD

Blend the strawberries in a food processor or blender to make a thick juice. Add the sweet almond oil and stir to mix well.

Apply to the face and neck and leave on for 10 minutes. Rinse off with bottled or spring water or a chamomile infusion, using cotton pads, and pat dry.

VARIATION

For those who are allergic to strawberries, try raspberries for a similar, but slightly less astringent, effect.

EFFECT	cleanses, tones
SKIN TYPES	normal, oily, combination; see VARIATION if allergic to strawberries.
FREQUENCY OF USE	once daily
SHELF LIFE	12 hours in refrigerator
PREPARATION TIME	5 minutes
TREATMENT TIME	10 minutes

oat and lemon juice mask

Anti-inflammatory oats and soothing almond oil complement lemon's citric acid in a robust, deep-cleansing, astringent mask. The mask's tonic action is especially good for preventing moisture loss in aging skin. For carrier oils, see pages 34 and 38; for hydrosols, see page 45; for infusions, see page 30.

INGREDIENTS

1 lemon (or orange for normal skin)
2 tablespoons sweet almond oil
4 tablespoons oatmeal flakes
witch hazel hydrosol (as required)
bottled or spring water
rose hydrosol

METHOD

Slice and press the lemon or orange to extract 3 tablespoons of juice. Stir the juice and sweet almond oil into the oatmeal flakes. Then gradually add enough witch hazel hydrosol to make a smooth paste, stirring all the time.

Apply evenly to the face and neck and leave on for 15 minutes. Rinse, using bottled or spring water and cotton pads, and pat dry. Dab on a little rose hydrosol, allowing to dry naturally.

VARIATIONS

For a more nourishing effect, substitute olive oil for sweet almond oil. Use an infusion of chamomile instead of witch hazel for a less astringent effect.

EFFECT	cleanses, tones, reduces inflammation
SKIN TYPES	all, especially aging
FREQUENCY OF USE	once a week
SHELF LIFE	12 hours in refrigerator
PREPARATION TIME	5 minutes
TREATMENT TIME	15 minutes

papaya exfoliating lotion

It is an enzyme called papain, most abundant in the flesh of the unripe papaya, that acts as an excellent mild exfoliant—literally digesting dead skin cells. The chamomile infusion should counteract the potential for inflammation. But if you have sensitive skin or are prone to allergic reactions, test first on your inside arm or wrist. Finishing with rose hydrosol rather than chamomile has a more toning effect. For infusions, see page 30; for hydrosols, see page 45.

INGREDIENTS
1 large fresh papaya
1 cup chamomile infusion, cooled
bottled or spring water
rose hydrosol (optional)

METHOD
Peel the papaya, remove the seeds, and purée the flesh in a food processor or blender. Press through a piece of muslin to extract all the juice. Mix the juice with an equal amount of chamomile infusion, stirring well.

Using cotton pads, apply the lotion to the face and neck, avoiding any contact with the eyes. Leave on for 10 minutes and rinse off with bottled or spring water. Dab on a little of the remaining chamomile infusion or some rose hydrosol and allow to dry naturally.
VARIATION
Dabbing with papaya juice is an excellent way to remove blackheads.

EFFECT	cleanses
SKIN TYPES	all, but test if sensitive or prone to allergic reactions
FREQUENCY OF USE	once a week
SHELF LIFE	12 hours in refrigerator
PREPARATION TIME	10 minutes
TREATMENT TIME	no more than 10 minutes

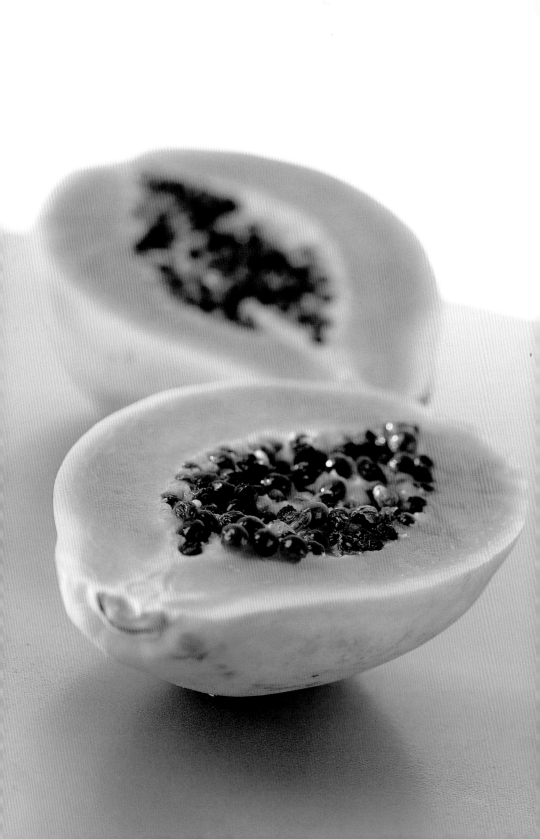

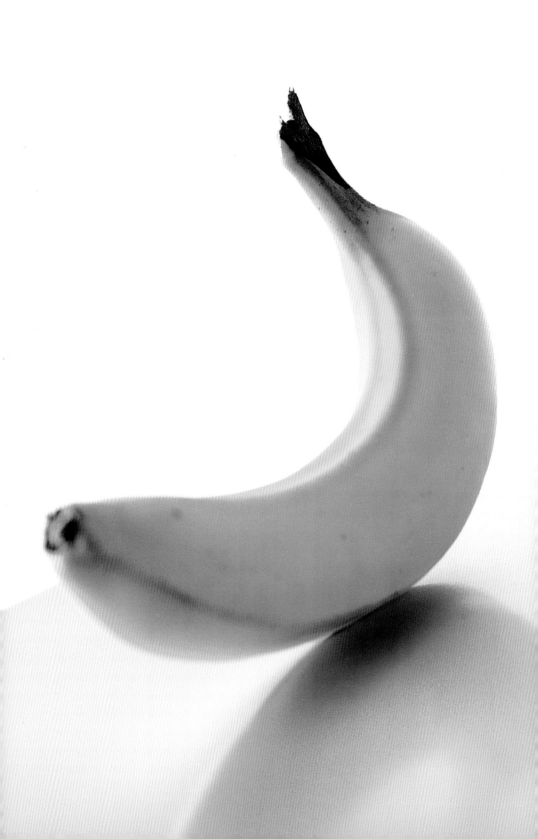

nourishing

recipes

banana anti-aging mask

Bananas are one of the most nourishing fruits available because they contain large quantities of magnesium, potassium, iron, zinc, iodine, and vitamins A, B (folic acid), E, and F. Here they are teamed with heavy cream (traditionally used to prevent wrinkles) and organic honey in a recipe crammed full of nutrients. For hydrosols, see page 45.

INGREDIENTS
1 small banana
2 tablespoons fresh heavy cream
1 tablespoon organic honey
1 tablespoon oat flour
bottled or spring water
rose hydrosol

METHOD
Mash the banana, using the back of a fork, and then add cream, honey, and flour. Stir to mix well. You may need to add a little more cream or flour to obtain the consistency of thick cream or yogurt.

Apply mask to the clean face, including the area around the eyes and the neck, and leave on for 30 minutes. Rinse off with bottled or spring water and cotton pads, and dab on a little rose hydrosol, allowing to dry naturally.

EFFECT	nourishes
SKIN TYPES	dry, aging
FREQUENCY OF USE	3 times a week
SHELF LIFE	6 hours in refrigerator
PREPARATION TIME	5 minutes
TREATMENT TIME	30 minutes

geranium oil and clay mask

This wonderfully scented mask derives its richness from the high vitamin E content in wheat germ oil and the linoleic acid (or vitamin F) in evening primrose oil, while geranium essential oil has a balancing, hydrating effect on the skin. Rosewood's gentle tonic action combines with the clay to make this recipe astringent as well as nourishing. For oils, see pages 34–41; for clay, see pages 22–24; for hydrosols, see page 45.

INGREDIENTS

1 tablespoon wheat germ oil
2 capsules 500I.U. evening primrose oil (contents only)
1 drop rosewood essential oil
1 drop geranium essential oil
3 tablespoons white or green clay powder
3 tablespoons rose hydrosol
bottled or spring water

METHOD

Blend the wheat germ and evening primrose carrier oils and then combine with the blended rosewood and geranium essential oils (see page 37). Add to the clay. Pour on the rose hydrosol and leave for 30 minutes before stirring. Mix well into a smooth paste.

For application to clean face and neck, see page 29 and leave on for 20 minutes. Remove with bottled or spring water and cotton pads.

EFFECT	nourishes, cleanses, tones, reduces inflammation
SKIN TYPES	all
FREQUENCY OF USE	once a week
SHELF LIFE	12 hours in refrigerator
PREPARATION TIME	5 minutes, plus 30 minutes "resting time"
TREATMENT TIME	20 minutes

spirulina vitalizing mask

The blue-green algae called spirulina are rich in beta-carotene and trace elements very beneficial to aging or damaged skin. You will find spirulina in powder form in most health-food shops. When applied daily, this mask is also effective in the treatment of acne. For clay, see pages 22–24; for carrier oils, see pages 34 and 38; for hydrosols, see page 45.

INGREDIENTS

1 tablespoon spirulina powder
2 tablespoons white or green clay powder
1 tablespoon olive oil
bottled or spring water
rose hydrosol

METHOD

Add the spirulina to the clay and stir in the olive oil. Pour on 3 table-spoons of bottled or spring water and set aside for 30 minutes without stirring. Then mix well to make a smooth paste.

For application to the clean face and neck, see page 29. Leave on for 20 minutes and then wash off with bottled or spring water, patting dry with cotton pads. Dab on a little rose hydrosol and allow to dry naturally.

VARIATION

Add 1 teaspoon of royal jelly (also available in health-food shops) to the smooth paste to boost the nourishing, vitalizing effect.

EFFECT	nourishes
SKIN TYPES	all
FREQUENCY OF USE	once a week
SHELF LIFE	8 hours in refrigerator
PREPARATION TIME	5 minutes, plus 30 minutes "resting time"
TREATMENT TIME	20 minutes

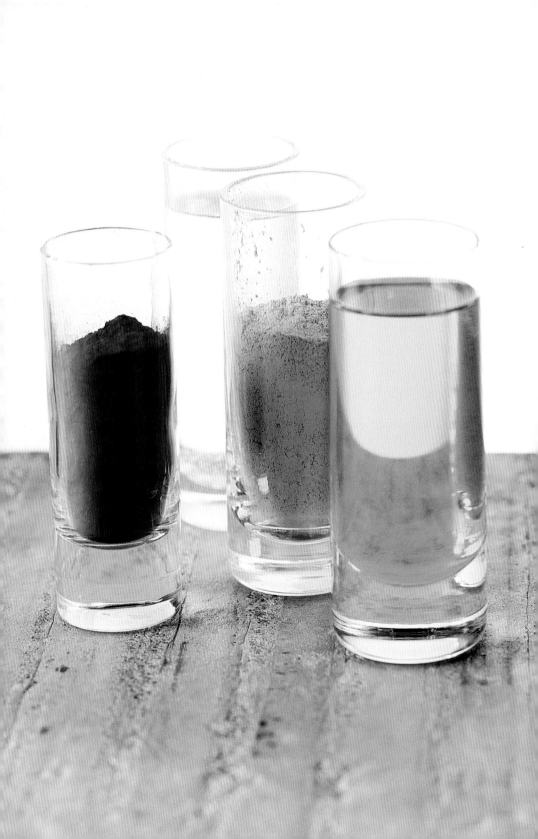

yogurt and carrot juice mask

This is an excellent mix for improving the elasticity of dry skin. The yogurt has a good balancing effect on the skin's pH. Carrot contains precious rejuvenating minerals, and honey's moistening action rejuvenates tired skin. For carrier oils, see pages 34 and 38; for hydrosols, see page 45.

INGREDIENTS

1 large carrot or 1 tablespoon carrot juice
2 tablespoons organic yogurt with live and active cultures
1 tablespoon sweet almond oil
1 tablespoon organic honey
bottled or spring water
rose hydrosol (optional)

METHOD

If making your own carrot juice, prepare 1 tablespoon. An alternative, if you don't have a juicer, is to use grated carrot, in which case you need 2 tablespoons. Mix the yogurt with the carrot, and stir in the sweet almond oil and honey.

Apply to the clean face and neck and leave on for 20 minutes. Rinse with bottled or spring water and pat dry. If you wish, finish with a dab of rose hydrosol and allow to dry naturally, .

VARIATION

Use wheat germ oil instead of sweet almond oil for an even more nourishing effect. Wheat germ contains vitamin E, which has a powerful healing, regenerative action.

EFFECT	nourishes, balances pH
SKIN TYPES	all, especially dry, aging, or damaged
FREQUENCY OF USE	once a week
SHELF LIFE	6 hours in refrigerator
PREPARATION TIME	5 minutes
TREATMENT TIME	20 minutes

fresh milk and lemon mask

You need fresh whole milk for this mask, which helps to balance the pH of dry or aging skin. The lemon juice is astringent, and therefore toning, but it also supplies a little vitamin C. For hydrosols, see page 45.

INGREDIENTS
½ **lemon**
9fl.oz (250ml) fresh whole milk
rose hydrosol

METHOD
Extract the juice of the half lemon and add to the milk, stirring to mix thoroughly.

Apply the resulting mixture to the clean face and neck, using cotton pads, and leave on to penetrate the skin for 20 minutes. When the skin is dry, clean gently, using rose hydrosol and cotton pads. Allow to dry naturally.

EFFECT	nourishes, cleanses, tones, balances pH
SKIN TYPES	all, especially dry or aging
FREQUENCY OF USE	once daily for 10 days
SHELF LIFE	6 hours in refrigerator
PREPARATION TIME	5 minutes
TREATMENT TIME	20 minutes

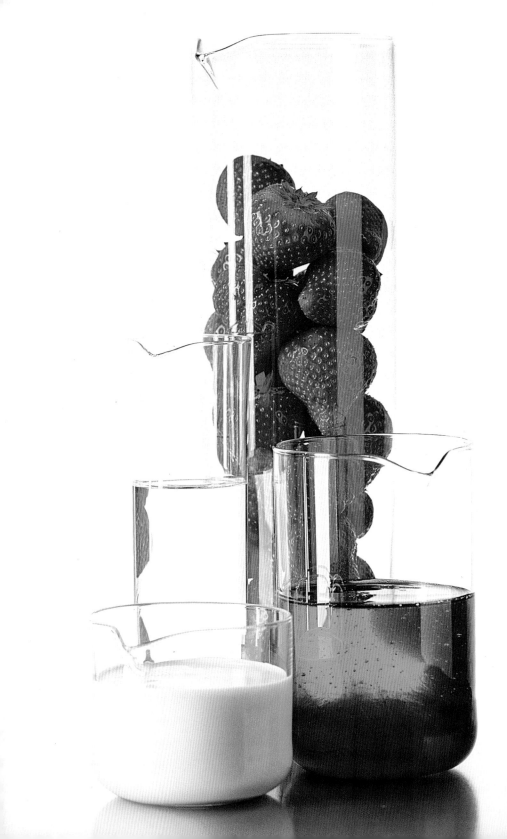

strawberry and cream mask

The honey, with its many trace elements, combines with the cream to nourish tired skin and keep it supple and moist. The salicylic acid in the strawberries cleanses by removing impurities and dead cells. If you have sensitive skin, see page 60. For hydrosols, see page 45.

INGREDIENTS
3–4 medium-sized, ripe strawberries
1 tablespoon fresh heavy cream
1 tablespoon organic honey
rose hydrosol

METHOD

Mash the strawberries with the back of a fork or purée them in a food processor or blender. Add the cream and honey to the purée to form a thick mixture. Add 1 teaspoon of clay if the mixture is too runny.

Apply to the clean face and neck, avoiding the area around the eyes, and leave on for 10 minutes. Rinse off, using bottled or spring water and cotton pads, and finish with a little rose hydrosol, allowing to dry naturally.

VARIATIONS

Substitute yogurt with live and active cultures for the cream to balance the pH of the skin. You can also use raspberries instead of strawberries. The yogurt/raspberry variation is suitable for sensitive skin, and it is also less likely to cause minor irritation for anyone allergic to strawberries.

EFFECT	nourishes, cleanses, balances pH if you substitute yogurt
SKIN TYPES	all (see VARIATION for sensitive skin)
FREQUENCY OF USE	once a week
SHELF LIFE	6 hours in refrigerator
PREPARATION TIME	2 minutes
TREATMENT TIME	10 minutes

pollen and egg yolk mask

Pollen and egg yolk are both rich in many of the vitamins, minerals, trace elements, and amino acids needed for healthy skin. This recipe is particularly beneficial if applied regularly to aging or damaged skin. For hydrosols, see page 45.

INGREDIENTS
1 tablespoon unprocessed pollen grains
2 large egg yolks
bottled or spring water
rose hydrosol

METHOD
Pulverize the pollen grains in a food processer or blender with just a few short bursts. You need a fine powder, but it is important to avoid heating the pollen because that destroys some of its active ingredients. Add the egg yolks, stirring well to mix.

Apply this mixture to the clean face and neck and leave on for 20 minutes. Rinse off with bottled or spring water, using cotton pads, and pat dry. Dab on a little rose hydrosol and allow to dry naturally.

VARIATION
You could use 2 tablespoons of fresh heavy cream instead of the egg yolks. The effect would be similar.

EFFECT	nourishes
SKIN TYPES	all, especially aging or damaged
FREQUENCY OF USE	once or twice a week
SHELF LIFE	6 hours in refrigerator
PREPARATION TIME	5 minutes
TREATMENT TIME	20 minutes

almond and egg white mask

Nourishing vitamins, fatty acids, trace elements, and enzymes in almond and honey combine with the astringent action of egg white to make a very effective mask for dry or aging skin. For hydrosols, see page 45.

INGREDIENTS
2oz (50g) whole almonds
1 large egg white
1 tablespoon organic honey
rose hydrosol (as required)
bottled or spring water

METHOD
Blanch the almonds in boiling water for 4 minutes and allow to cool. Beat the egg white lightly. Peel the almonds and give them a quick grind in a blender or coffee grinder until you have a coarse granular texture. Add the lightly beaten egg white and the honey, and blend again to form a smooth paste. If the consistency is too thick to spread easily, stir in some rose hydrosol, a little at a time.

Apply evenly to the clean face and neck and leave on for 20 minutes. Rinse with bottled or spring water, using cotton pads, and pat dry. Dab on a little rose hydrosol and allow to dry naturally.

VARIATIONS
Ground almonds would shorten the preparation time (do not blanch). Finish with a half-and-half mixture of rose hydrosol and witch hazel (see page 62) for a more toning action.

EFFECT	nourishes
SKIN TYPES	dry, aging
FREQUENCY OF USE	once daily
SHELF LIFE	6 hours in refrigerator
PREPARATION TIME	5 minutes
TREATMENT TIME	20 minutes

honey and egg yolk mask

Egg yolk contains vitamins A, D, and E, plus essential amino acids, minerals, and trace elements, in a form that the skin can easily absorb and process. Here it is paired with moisturizing honey in a recipe that is an excellent boost for any kind of tired skin. For clay, see pages 22–24; for hydrosols, see page 45.

INGREDIENTS
1 tablespoon organic honey
1 large egg yolk
1 teaspoon white or green clay powder or oat flour
bottled or spring water
rose hydrosol

METHOD
Combine the honey, egg yolk, and clay or oat flour, stirring to create a fine paste.

Apply evenly to the clean face and neck and leave on for 20 minutes. Rinse off with bottled or spring water, using cotton pads, and pat dry. Dab on a little rose hydrosol and allow to dry naturally.

EFFECT	nourishes
SKIN TYPES	all, especially dry or aging
FREQUENCY OF USE	2 or 3 times a week for dry or aging skin; once every 2 weeks for all others
SHELF LIFE	6 hours in refrigerator
PREPARATION TIME	5 minutes
TREATMENT TIME	20 minutes

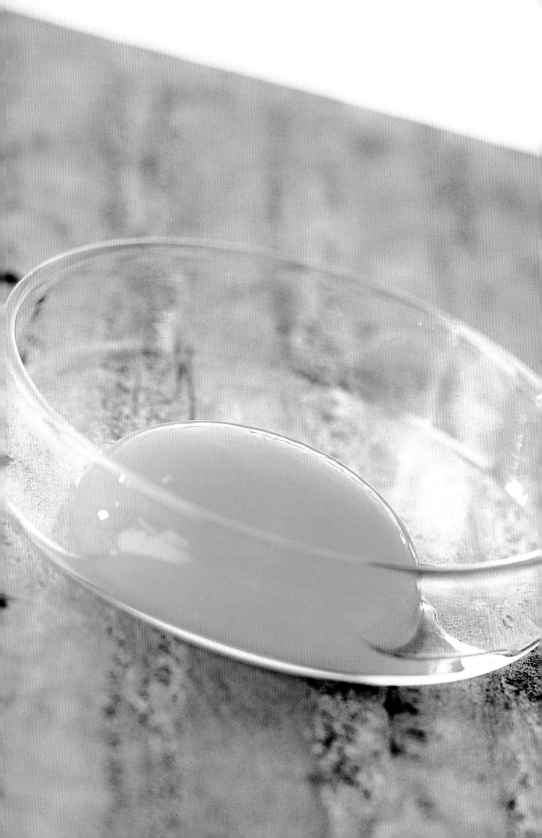

fresh parsley mask

Fresh parsley adds vitamins A, B, and C and iron to this toning and nourishing mask, which is particularly good for the neck. Choose heavy cream for a more nourishing effect on dry skin, yogurt for other skin types. For oils, see pages 38–39; for hydrosols, see page 45.

INGREDIENTS

1 small bunch fresh parsley
3 tablespoons fresh heavy cream or organic yogurt with live and active cultures
1 tablespoon organic honey
2 capsules 500I.U. evening primrose oil (contents only)
bottled or spring water
rose hydrosol

METHOD

Clean the parsley in cold water and remove as much of the stalks as possible. Chop the leaves fine by hand or using a food processor or blender. Add the heavy cream or yogurt and the honey and evening primrose oil. Stir or blend to mix well.

Apply evenly to the clean face and neck and leave on for 20 minutes. Rinse, using bottled or spring water and cotton pads, and pat dry. Apply a little rose hydrosol and allow to dry naturally.

VARIATIONS

For dry, scaly eczema, use 2 capsules of borage oil instead of primrose oil. For a much stronger anti-inflammatory action, substitute watercress for the parsley.

EFFECT	nourishes, cleanses, tones, reduces inflammation
SKIN TYPES	all, especially aging
FREQUENCY OF USE	once a week
SHELF LIFE	6 hours in refrigerator
PREPARATION TIME	10 minutes
TREATMENT TIME	20 minutes

avocado and cream mask

This extremely rich mask is packed full of vitamins: Avocados alone contain A, B, and C, plus essential amino acids. For carrier oils, see pages 34 and 38; for hydrosols, see page 45.

INGREDIENTS

½ **very ripe avocado, pitted**

2 tablespoons fresh heavy cream

1 tablespoon wheat germ oil

3 capsules 500I.U. evening primrose (contents only)

bottled or spring water

rose hydrosol

METHOD

Peel the halved avocado and mash the flesh with the back of a fork. Discard the avocado pit. Add the heavy cream, wheat germ oil, and evening primrose oil, stirring well to mix.

Apply evenly to clean face and neck and leave on for 20 minutes. Rinse with bottled or spring water and cotton pads and pat dry. Dab on a little rose hydrosol and allow to dry naturally.

VARIATION

Substitute 3 capsules of borage oil for evening primrose oil to produce a similar but more potent effect.

EFFECT	nourishes
SKIN TYPES	dry, aging
FREQUENCY OF USE	twice a week for dry skin; daily for aging skin
SHELF LIFE	6 hours in refrigerator
PREPARATION TIME	5 minutes
TREATMENT TIME	20 minutes

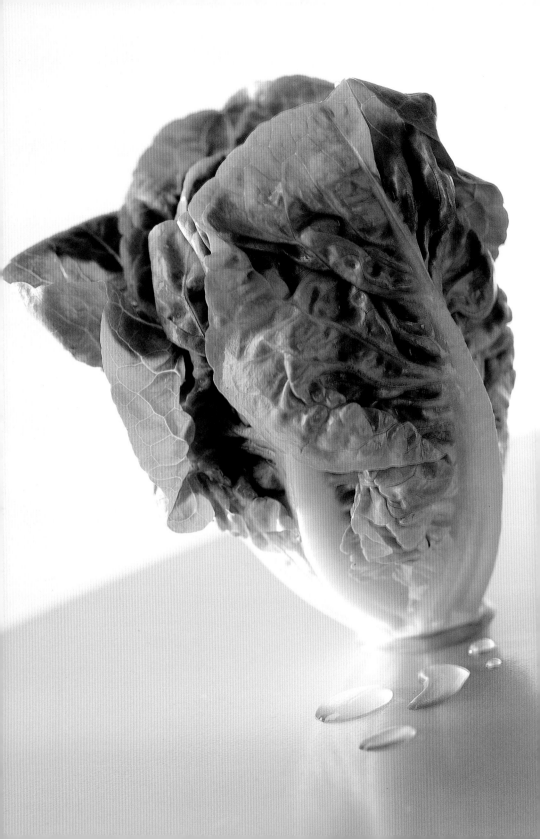

lettuce leaf mask

Cooling and anti-inflammatory, lettuce leaves calm skin rashes and sunburn rapidly, while their vitamins (A, C, D, E, and F), precious minerals, and trace elements hydrate as well as nourish.

INGREDIENTS

1 very fresh small head of lettuce, preferably organic

METHOD

Separate the leaves of the lettuce and clean. Toss into boiling water for 5 minutes until cooked. Drain quickly, reserving both leaves and liquid, and allow to cool. The cooking water can be stored in a covered container in the refrigerator and used as a lotion for the face and neck.

Carefully apply cooled leaves to clean face and neck and leave in place for 5–10 minutes, if possible; they will be rather slippery! Pat the face dry with cotton pads.

VARIATION

Purée the cooked lettuce leaves in a food processor or blender. Into the purée stir 3 tablespoons of white or green clay and 1 tablespoon of fresh carrot juice; then add 2 tablespoons of the lettuce cooking water and set aside without stirring for 30 minutes. Mix well to form a smooth paste. Apply evenly to the clean face and neck and leave on for 20 minutes, rinsing off with bottled or spring water. This makes an excellent mask for dry or aging skin that suffers from inflammation or dry eczema.

EFFECT	nourishes, hydrates, reduces inflammation
SKIN TYPES	dry, damaged (see also VARIATION)
FREQUENCY OF USE	once daily
SHELF LIFE	cooked leaves: 12 hours in refrigerator; cooking water: 3 days in refrigerator
PREPARATION TIME	10 minutes; VARIATION 10 minutes, plus 30 minutes "resting time"
TREATMENT TIME	10 minutes; VARIATION 20 minutes

high nutrient and vitamin mask

Carrot's high vitamin and mineral content—vitamins A and B (folic acid), plus iron, potassium, magnesium, manganese, sulphur, and copper—make it an important vegetable in skin care. Here it is teamed with vitamin E (in the wheat germ) and nourishing honey and yogurt in a mask most suitable for those with dry or aging skin but which can be used occasionally on all skin types. For carrier oils, see pages 34 and 38; for clay, see pages 22–24; for hydrosols, see pages 14–19 and 45.

INGREDIENTS

1 large carrot or 2 tablespoons carrot juice
5 tablespoons wheat germ oil
2 tablespoons organic honey
2 tablespoons organic yogurt with live and active cultures
1 teaspoon oat flour or clay powder (as necessary)
bottled or spring water

METHOD

If making your own carrot juice, prepare 2 tablespoons. Combine the wheat germ oil, honey, yogurt, and carrot juice, stirring well. Adjust the consistency by adding a little more wheat germ oil or carrot juice if too thick, or clay or oat flour if too runny.

Apply evenly to the clean face and neck and leave on for 20 minutes. Rinse with bottled or spring water and cotton pads and pat dry. Dab on a suitable hydrosol and allow to dry naturally.

EFFECT	nourishes, balances pH
SKIN TYPES	all
FREQUENCY OF USE	daily for aging or damaged skin; once a week for dry skin; 3–4 weeks for other skin types
SHELF LIFE	6 hours in refrigerator
PREPARATION TIME	5 minutes
TREATMENT TIME	20 minutes

healing mask

These blended oils make a excellent mask to apply daily for a few weeks on aging or damaged skin, but dry or sensitive skin will benefit too. This quantity will last for about two weeks. For oils, see pages 34–41.

INGREDIENTS

4 teaspoons wheat germ oil
4 teaspoons rosehip oil
6 capsules 500I.U. evening primrose oil (contents only)
5 drops geranium essential oil
bottled or spring water

METHOD

Pour the wheat germ, rosehip, and evening primrose oils into a 50ml brown bottle (see page 37) and then add the geranium essential oil. Close the bottle and shake well.

Twice a day, dampen the clean face and neck lightly with bottled or spring water and, using a piece of cotton, apply a little oil to the entire surface, including the areas around the eyes. Add a little more in any areas that are particularly wrinkled or dry. Don't be overgenerous—only a slight oily film should be left on the skin. Leave it on to be absorbed in its own time—it will take 20 minutes. Makeup can be applied as soon as the oil has disappeared.

VARIATION

Substitute borage oil for evening primrose oil. Its effect is more potent.

EFFECT	nourishes
SKIN TYPES	aging, damaged, dry, sensitive
FREQUENCY OF USE	twice daily
SHELF LIFE	1 month
PREPARATION TIME	5 minutes
TREATMENT TIME	20 minutes

yogurt and evening primrose mask

Vitamin E and the gamma linoleic acid (or polyunsaturated fatty acid) in evening primrose oil feature strongly in a revitalizing mix that must be used for several weeks for best results. For carrier oils, see pages 34 and 38; for clay, see pages 22–24; for hydrosols, see page 45.

INGREDIENTS

3 tablespoons yogurt with live and active cultures
2 capsules 500I.U. evening primrose oil (contents only)
1 teaspoon organic honey
2 capsules 400I.U. vitamin E oil (contents only)
white or green clay powder or oat flour (as necessary)
bottled or spring water
rose hydrosol

METHOD

Mix all the ingredients together, stirring well. If the consistency is too runny, add a little clay or flour and stir again.

Apply evenly to the clean face and neck and leave on for 20 minutes. Rinse off, using bottled or spring water and cotton pads, and pat dry. Tone the skin by dabbing on a little rose hydrosol, and allow to dry naturally.

VARIATIONS

Substitute 2 capsules of borage oil for the evening primrose oil and/or 1 teaspoon of wheat germ oil for the vitamin E. Borage oil is more potent than evening primrose oil; wheat germ contains less vitamin E.

EFFECT	nourishes, balances pH, reduces inflammation
SKIN TYPES	all, especially dry or aging
FREQUENCY OF USE	twice a week or more for aging skin; occasionally for all others
SHELF LIFE	6 hours in refrigerator
PREPARATION TIME	5 minutes
TREATMENT TIME	20 minutes

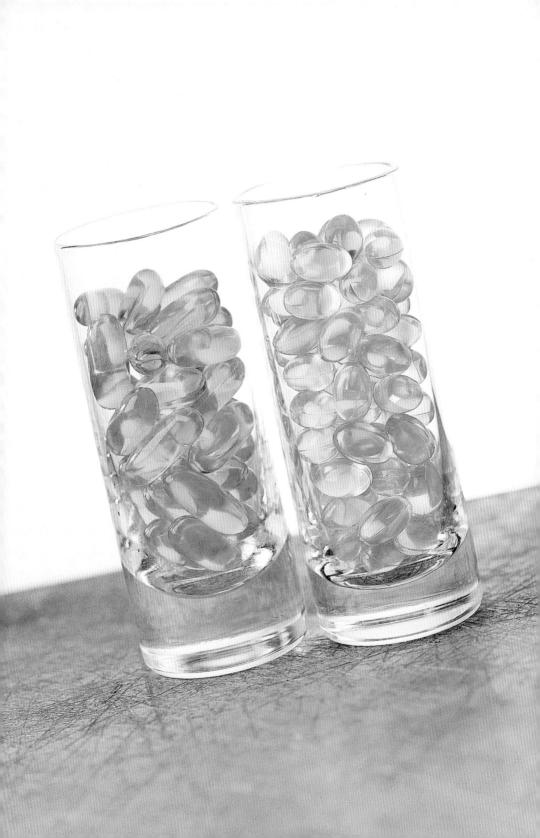

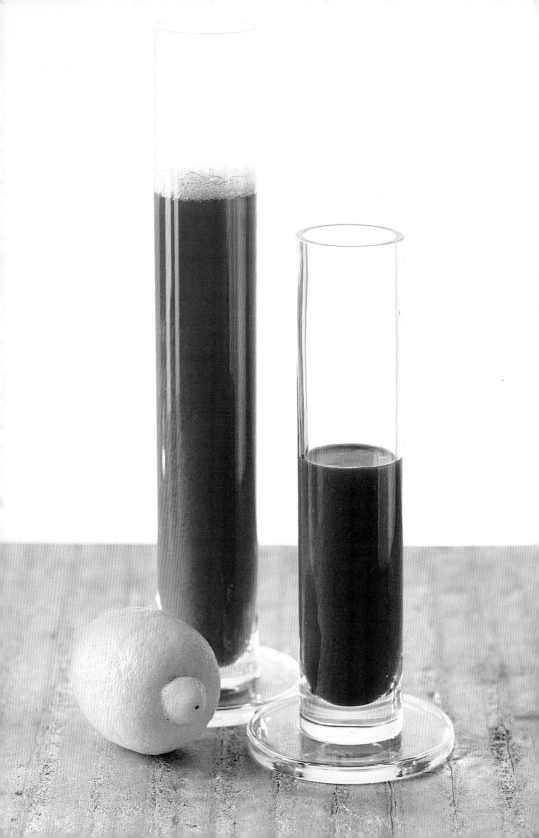

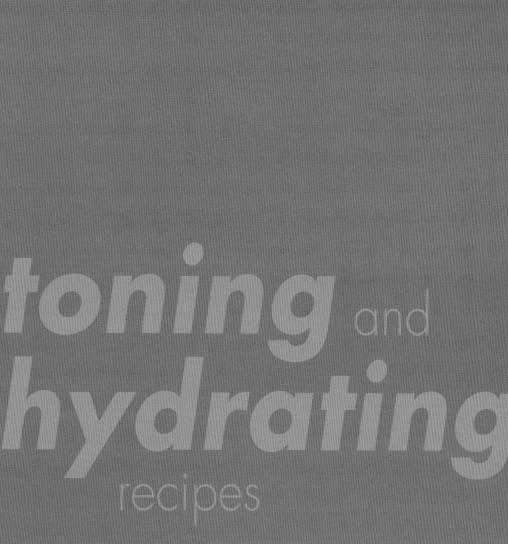

toning and

hydrating

recipes

cucumber and fresh mint mask

The fresh mint and egg white both have a toning action on the skin, while the cucumber is hydrating and anti-inflammatory, making this a mask that can also be used to calm inflamed skin or sunburn.

INGREDIENTS

5 fresh mint leaves
¼ medium cucumber
1 large egg white
bottled or spring water

METHOD

Place the mint in a food processor or blender and give it one short burst to chop. Peel and seed the cucumber. Add to the mint in the processor or blender and purée. Beat the egg separately until it stands in stiff peaks. Fold it very gently into the puréed cucumber mixture.

Apply evenly to the face and neck and leave on for 20 minutes. Rinse off, using bottled or spring water and cotton pads, and pat dry.

VARIATIONS

For an even more toning effect, add 1 teaspoon of freshly squeezed lemon juice or apple cider vinegar. Trickle slowly into the final mixture, stirring gently all the time.

EFFECT	tones, hydrates, reduces inflammation
SKIN TYPES	all
FREQUENCY OF USE	once a week
SHELF LIFE	6 hours in refrigerator
PREPARATION TIME	10 minutes
TREATMENT TIME	20 minutes

apple juice and clay mask

Substituting fresh apple juice for water in a clay mask creates a more toning preparation for the face and neck. Nourishing wheat germ counteracts the drying effect of clay on a dry or aging skin. For carrier oils, see pages 34 and 38; for clay, see pages 22–24; for hydrosols, see page 45.

INGREDIENTS

1–2 apples or 3 tablespoons fresh apple juice
1 tablespoon wheat germ oil
2 tablespoons white or green clay powder
bottled or spring water
rose hydrosol

METHOD

If making your own apple juice, extract 3 tablespoons, using a juicer. Following the clay mask method (see pages 23–24), stir the wheat germ oil into the clay and pour on the apple juice. Set aside for 30 minutes before stirring to form a smooth paste.

For application to the face and neck and removal, see page 29. Finish with a little rose hydrosol.

EFFECT	tones, cleanses, reduces inflammation
SKIN TYPES	all
FREQUENCY OF USE	once or twice a week
SHELF LIFE	8 hours in refrigerator
PREPARATION TIME	5 minutes, plus 30 minutes "resting time"
TREATMENT TIME	20 minutes

egg white and lemon juice mask

This classic recipe is probably still the best toner around, judged for its simplicity and remarkable effectiveness. It is also an excellent treatment for softening the skin of the hands. Egg white's ability to remove impurities and lemon juice's action in inhibiting bacterial growth explain this mask's subsidiary cleansing action. For hydrosols, see page 45.

INGREDIENTS
1 large egg white
½ lemon
bottled or spring water
rose or witch hazel hydrosol

METHOD
Beat the egg white stiffly until it stands up in peaks and press the half lemon to extract 1 teaspoon of juice. Then simply fold the juice carefully into the egg white.

Apply to the face and neck and leave on for 20 minutes. Rinse off, using bottled or spring water and cotton pads, and pat dry. Dab on a little rose or witch hazel and allow to dry naturally.

EFFECT	tones, cleanses, nourishes
SKIN TYPES	all
FREQUENCY OF USE	twice a week for aging skin; once a week for all others
SHELF LIFE	6 hours in refrigerator
PREPARATION TIME	5 minutes
TREATMENT TIME	20 minutes

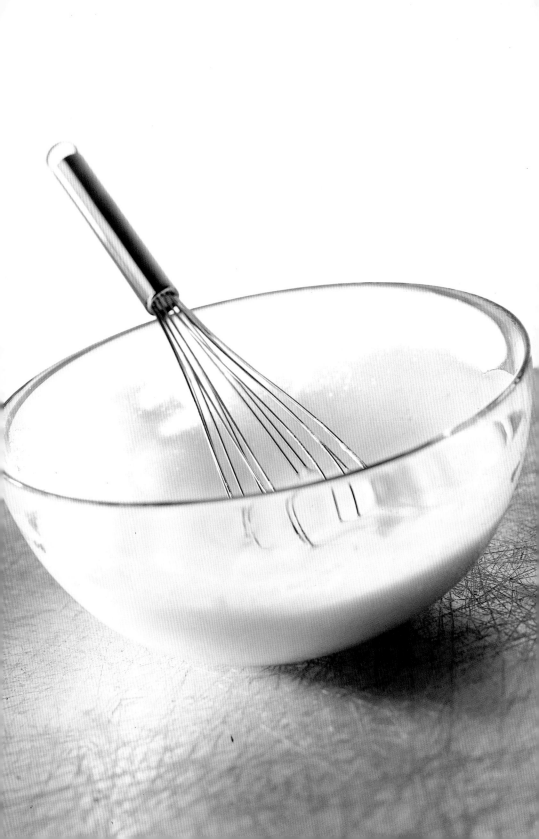

fresh parsley and clay mask

Here astringent witch hazel combines with anti-aging agents in the fresh parsley and olive oil to make this mask an excellent way to tone and nourish the skin of the neck. It can also be applied to the face, but take care to avoid the eyes. For clay, see pages 22–24; for carrier oils, see pages 34 and 38; for hydrosols, see page 45.

INGREDIENTS
small bunch fresh parsley
2 tablespoons white or green clay powder
3 tablespoons extra virgin olive oil
2 tablespoons witch hazel hydrosol
bottled or spring water

METHOD
Wash the parsley in cold water and remove the stalks before chopping the leaves fine by hand or using a food processor or blender. Stir 2 tablespoons of chopped parsley into the clay. Then add the olive oil and witch hazel, and stir again until a thick paste is obtained.

Apply to the neck and jawline and leave on for 20 minutes. Rinse off, using bottled or spring water and cotton pads, and pat dry.

VARIATION
Substitute wheat germ oil for the olive oil if you want the healing, regenerative effect of vitamin E.

EFFECT	tones, nourishes, reduces inflammation
SKIN TYPES	all
FREQUENCY OF USE	once a week
SHELF LIFE	12 hours in refrigerator
PREPARATION TIME	5 minutes
TREATMENT TIME	20 minutes

yogurt and blackcurrant mask

The fruit acid in blackcurrants is toning, hydrating, cleansing, and anti-inflammatory. When complemented with the balancing action of live yogurt, it creates a mask particularly beneficial for aging, flushed, or inflamed skin. Blackcurrants are also rich in trace elements, minerals (calcium, potassium and magnesium), and vitamins B and C. Use fresh fruit if available, although frozen blackcurrants are acceptable. Avoid canned fruit—it is heated in the preservation process, and the juice takes on the properties of purple dye. Removable but hardly relaxing!

INGREDIENTS
4 tablespoons blackcurrants
2 tablespoons yogurt with live and active cultures
bottled or spring water

METHOD
Crush the blackcurrants in a food processor or blender. Add the yogurt to the thick juice and stir well.

Apply to the face and neck and leave on for 20 minutes. Rinse off, using bottled or spring water and cotton pads, and pat dry.

EFFECT	tones, cleanses, hydrates, balances pH, reduces inflammation
SKIN TYPES	all, especially aging
FREQUENCY OF USE	twice a week
SHELF LIFE	6 hours in refrigerator
PREPARATION TIME	5 minutes
TREATMENT TIME	20 minutes

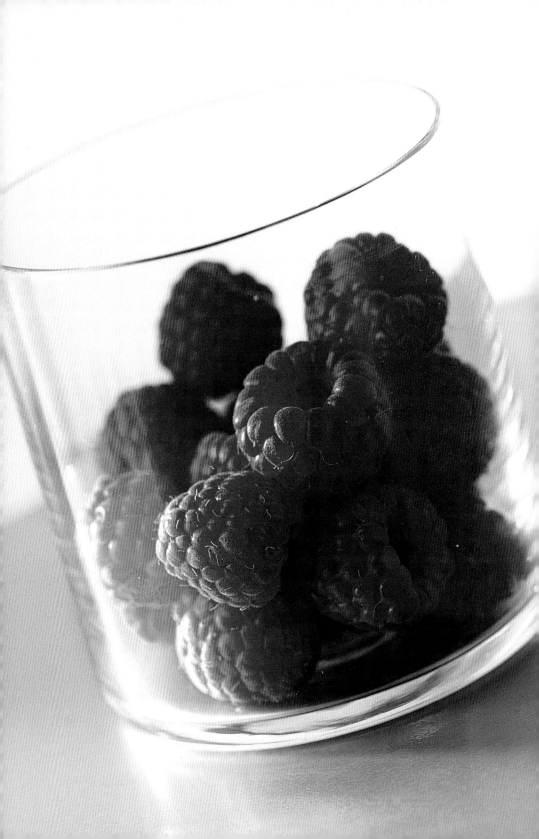

raspberry mask

The three fruit acids (salicylic, citric, and malic) in raspberries and the lactic acid in the milk combine for a more astringent, invigorating effect than that produced by the blackcurrant mask on page 99. For essential oils, see pages 34 and 40; for hydrosols, see page 45.

INGREDIENTS
12 raspberries
2 tablespoons fresh whole milk
1 drop geranium essential oil
bottled or spring water
witch hazel hydrosol

METHOD
Using a blender, food processor, or fork, crush enough raspberries to obtain 2 tablespoons of purée. Add to it the milk and geranium essential oil, and stir to mix well.

Apply to the face and neck, using cotton pads, and leave on for 20 minutes. Rinse, using bottled or spring water and more cotton pads, and pat dry. Finish by dabbing on a little witch hazel and allow to dry naturally.

VARIATION
For a more balancing effect, substitute yogurt with live and active cultures for the whole milk.

EFFECT	tones, hydrates, cleanses, reduces inflammation
SKIN TYPES	dry, combination, and especially aging
FREQUENCY OF USE	twice a week
SHELF LIFE	6 hours in refrigerator
PREPARATION TIME	5 minutes
TREATMENT TIME	20 minutes

egg white and cucumber mask

This cooling mask is excellent for dry, flushed, or inflamed skin. Both the egg white and the orange juice have a tonic action, while cucumber is hydrating and anti-inflammatory. Cucumber also contains vitamins A, B, and C; sulphur; manganese; and iodine. For hydrosols, see page 45.

INGREDIENTS
1 large egg white
½ orange
¼ cucumber
bottled or spring water
witch hazel or rose hydrosol

METHOD
Beat an egg white until it forms stiff peaks. Press the half orange to extract 1 tablespoon of juice. Grate enough cucumber to fill 2 tablespoons. Fold the cucumber carefully into the beaten egg white and add the orange juice, stirring gently to mix.

Apply to the face and neck and leave on for 20 minutes. Rinse with bottled or spring water and cotton pads. Then dab on a little witch hazel or rose hydrosol and allow to dry naturally.

EFFECT	tones, cleanses, hydrates, reduces inflammation
SKIN TYPES	dry, combination, aging, damaged
FREQUENCY OF USE	once or twice a week
SHELF LIFE	6 hours in refrigerator
PREPARATION TIME	5 minutes
TREATMENT TIME	20 minutes

fresh cream and grape lotion

Grapes are rich in minerals (potassium, manganese, calcium, sodium, and iodine) and vitamins A, B, and C. Black grapes also contain the bioflavonoid quercinine, a powerful antioxidant with an anti-aging action, so opt for those wherever possible. In this recipe grape and lemon juice act as toners, while the nourishing heavy cream counterbalances their astringent effect. For hydrosols, see page 45.

INGREDIENTS
several grapes or 1 tablespoon grape juice
½ lemon
1 tablespoon fresh heavy cream
bottled or spring water
witch hazel hydrosol

METHOD

If making your own grape juice, crush the grapes with a fork and press through a strainer to extract 1 tablespoon of juice. Press the lemon to extract half a teaspoon of juice. Beat the heavy cream and grape juice together to obtain a light, fluffy cream. Add the lemon juice gradually drop by drop to prevent curdling, stirring gently to mix well.

Apply to the face and neck and leave on for 10 minutes. Rinse, using bottled or spring water and cotton pads. To finish, dab on a little witch hazel and allow to dry naturally.

EFFECT	tones, nourishes
SKIN TYPES	all
FREQUENCY OF USE	once a week
SHELF LIFE	6 hours in refrigerator
PREPARATION TIME	5 minutes
TREATMENT TIME	10 minutes

apple cologne

The malic acid in fresh apple juice is mildly toning, is astringent, and helps to keep the skin clear, making this recipe suitable even for sensitive skin. It will keep for weeks because of its high alcohol content and is therefore useful when traveling.

INGREDIENTS

3–4 apples or 3½fl.oz (100ml) fresh apple juice

1 teaspoon sea salt

1 tablespoon organic honey

4 tablespoons good-quality European eau de cologne
or aftershave, or 100-proof vodka

METHOD

If making your own apple juice, prepare and filter through a paper towel. Discard the pulp. To the juice, add the sea salt, honey, and eau de cologne, aftershave, or vodka. Pour into a bottle, cover, and shake well to mix.

Use twice a day, applying to the face and neck with a cotton pad and allowing to dry naturally.

VARIATION

You can substitute filtered grape juice (see page 103) for the apple juice; the effect will be similar.

EFFECT	tones, hydrates, cleanses, nourishes
SKIN TYPES	all
FREQUENCY OF USE	twice daily
SHELF LIFE	1 month
PREPARATION TIME	5 minutes
TREATMENT TIME	20 minutes

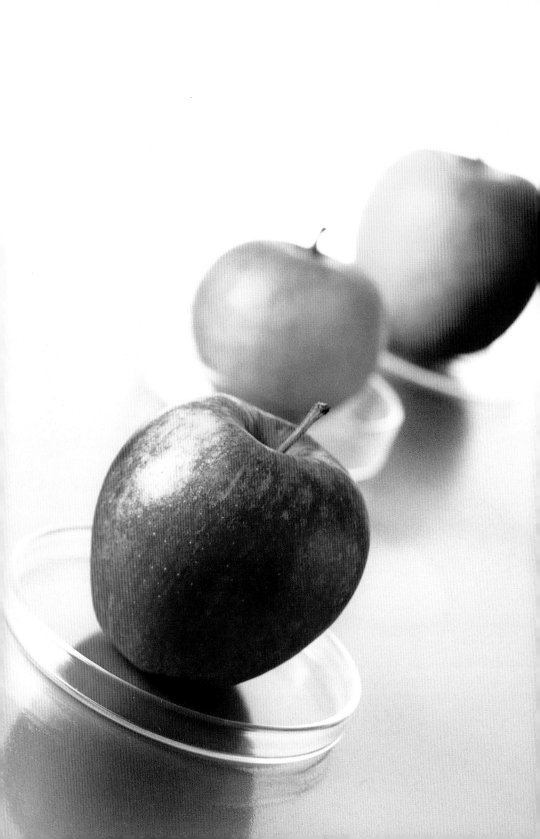

rose hydrosol astringent lotion

The combination of lemon juice, rose hydrosol, and witch hazel makes for an astringent toner that needs moisturizing, nourishing honey to keep it balanced. Like the previous recipe, this one is a useful traveling companion. Choose aftershave if you want to enhance the soothing action. For hydrosols, see page 45.

INGREDIENTS

½ **lemon**
3½ **tablespoons rose hydrosol**
3½ **tablespoons witch hazel hydrosol**
1 **tablespoon organic honey**
2fl.oz (50ml) **European eau de cologne or aftershave,
        or 100-proof vodka**

METHOD

Press the half lemon to extract 1 teaspoon of juice. Combine the rose and witch hazel, and then add the honey, lemon juice, and eau de cologne, aftershave, or vodka, stirring well. Pour into a bottle and cover to store.

Use twice a day, applying to the face and neck with cotton pads and allowing to dry naturally.

EFFECT	tones
SKIN TYPES	all
FREQUENCY OF USE	twice daily
SHELF LIFE	1 month
PREPARATION TIME	5 minutes
TREATMENT TIME	20 minutes

cucumber and vinegar lotion

It is the cucumber that hydrates and reduces inflammation. Vinegar and vodka are essentially toners here. This is a speedy recipe if you have apple cider vinegar at hand. If you don't, turn to page 46 for a description of this vinegar's properties and how to make it. Incidentally, this is not an opportunity to get rid of that bottle of malt vinegar lurking in your store cupboard. You must use good-quality white wine or cider vinegar.

INGREDIENTS
½ **cucumber**
apple cider vinegar
2 tablespoons 100-proof vodka

METHOD
Peel and seed the cucumber. Using a food processor or blender, process the flesh. Extract and reserve all the juice by straining through a piece of muslin. Discard the pulp. Add to the cucumber juice an equal amount of apple cider vinegar, and then the vodka, and stir well. Store in a closed bottle in the refrigerator.

Use twice a day, applying to the face and neck with cotton pads and allowing to dry naturally.

EFFECT	tones, hydrates, reduces inflammation
SKIN TYPES	all
FREQUENCY OF USE	twice daily
SHELF LIFE	2 weeks in refrigerator
PREPARATION TIME	10 minutes
TREATMENT TIME	20 minutes

barley and rosemary lotion

Rosemary tones, improving blood circulation in the skin. Barley water is a mild cleanser with some nourishing properties: Barley contains vitamins B and E and essential minerals (iodine, potassium, calcium, magnesium, iron, and copper). Soaking the barley for 24 hours is not essential, but it causes the grain to germinate, releasing a variety of enzymes that constitute an exfoliant gentle enough for sensitive skin.

INGREDIENTS
3½oz (100g) barley
2pt (1 liter) water
generous handful fresh rosemary or 3 tablespoons dried rosemary

METHOD
Cover the barley with cold water and set aside it to soak for 24 hours. Reserving the barley, strain off the soaking water. Cook the pre-soaked barley in 2 pints (1 liter) of fresh water for 30 minutes, bringing it to a boil, covering, and then leaving to simmer. Strain immediately, discarding the barley. Add the rosemary to the cooking water, covering and leaving to infuse until cool. Strain the liquid again and store in a closed bottle in the refrigerator.

Using cotton pads, apply twice a day to the face and neck and allow to dry naturally.

EFFECT	tones, cleanses, nourishes, reduces inflammation
SKIN TYPES	all
FREQUENCY OF USE	twice daily
SHELF LIFE	4 days in refrigerator
PREPARATION TIME	40 minutes, plus optional 24-hour "soaking time"
TREATMENT TIME	20 minutes

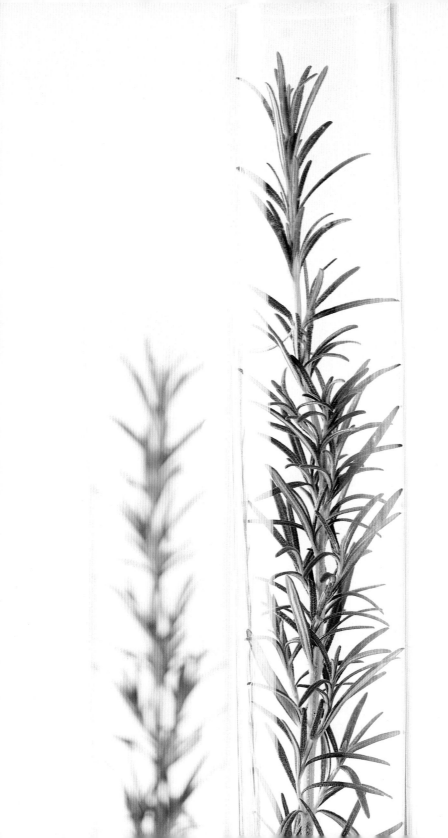

fresh juice toner

This recipe depends for best results on very fresh ingredients. Here highly astringent lemon plays the minor role in a mix of toning fruit acids. For advice on blackcurrants, see page 99; for grapes, see page 103.

INGREDIENTS

½ cup blackcurrants

10 grapes or 3fl.oz (75ml) fresh grape juice

½ lemon

METHOD

Crush the blackcurrants in a food processor or blender and strain through a piece of muslin, reserving the juice—you need 2⅗fl.oz. Repeat with the grapes if making your own grape juice. Press the half lemon to extract 1 tablespoon of juice. Pour the grape juice and blackcurrant juice into a bottle and add the lemon juice. Cover and store in the refrigerator.

Apply to the face and neck twice a day, using cotton pads, and allow to dry naturally.

EFFECT	tones, hydrates
SKIN TYPES	all
FREQUENCY OF USE	twice daily
SHELF LIFE	48 hours in refrigerator
PREPARATION TIME	10 minutes
TREATMENT TIME	20 minutes

rose, honey, and lemon lotion

This recipe combines the toning effect of rose, the nourishing qualities of honey, and the potent astringent action of lemon juice. Multiply the quantities given by five and you have enough for a week. For hydrosols, see page 45.

INGREDIENTS

½ **lemon**

2 tablespoons rose hydrosol

1 teaspoon organic honey

METHOD

Press the half lemon to extract the juice and mix with the rose and honey, stirring well.

Apply daily to the face and neck, using cotton pads, and allow to dry naturally.

EFFECT	tones, hydrates, nourishes, cleanses
SKIN TYPES	all
FREQUENCY OF USE	once daily
SHELF LIFE	1 week in refrigerator
PREPARATION TIME	2 minutes
TREATMENT TIME	20 minutes

fresh melon lotion

Primarily composed of water, natural sugars, and small amounts of vitamins A, B, and C, melons are cooling and hydrating. Indeed, used alone, crushed melon flesh will quickly calm the pain of a mild burn or sunburn. Lemon, the toner, and olive oil are complementary and work together to balance the pH of the skin. For carrier oils, see pages 34 and 38.

INGREDIENTS
¼ **fresh, ripe melon (any variety)**
½ **lemon**
1 tablespoon olive oil

METHOD
Peel and seed the melon. Press the half lemon to extract 1 teaspoon of lemon juice. Using a food processor or blender, purée the fresh melon. Filter its juice through a piece of muslin and reserve. Add to the melon juice the olive oil and lemon juice, and store in a covered bottle or container in the refrigerator.

Shake well before use. Apply twice a day to the face and neck, using cotton pads, and allow to dry naturally.

VARIATIONS
For a longer lasting but less hydrating preparation, add 2 tablespoons of good-quality European eau de cologne, aftershave, or 100-proof vodka after the lemon juice.

EFFECT	tones, hydrates, reduces inflammation
SKIN TYPES	all
FREQUENCY OF USE	twice daily
SHELF LIFE	in refrigerator: BASIC RECIPE 48 hours; VARIATIONS: 2 weeks
PREPARATION TIME	10 minutes
TREATMENT TIME	20 minutes

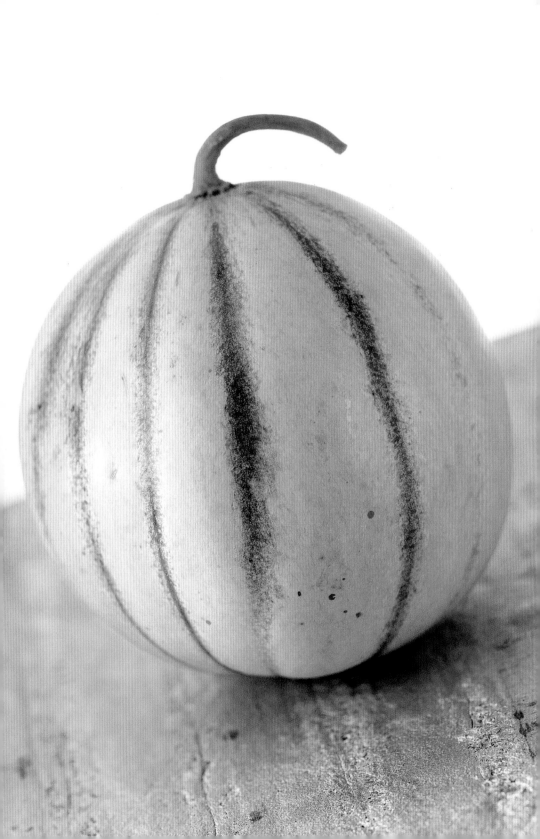

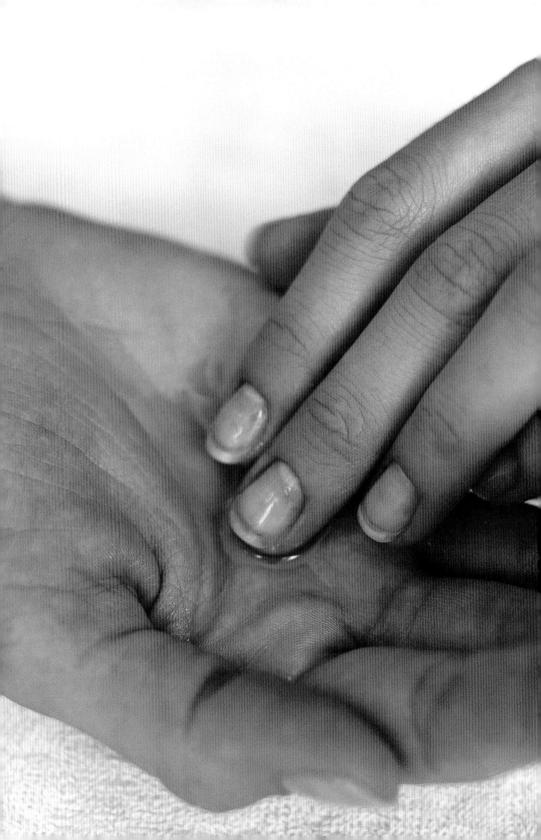

treating
skin
problems

acne

This very common condition affects more females than males. Although it starts in, and is often associated with, teenagers, it can recur for years, sometimes right through to middle age. The characteristic small fatty lumps—actually swollen sebaceous glands (see page 6)—are frequently inflamed and topped with black or white heads that, if squeezed, can set off a cycle of re-infection due to bacterial activity on the surface of the skin. When the lumps do finally subside, some scarring is almost inevitable. The face is most likely to be affected, but acne can also appear on the neck, shoulders, back, and upper chest.

Acne occurs in people whose sebaceous glands are particularly sensitive to testosterone. Known as the male hormone, testosterone is in fact produced in varying amounts by both sexes. Medical research has revealed that there is an increased amount of testosterone in a woman's skin at the end of each menstrual cycle, prior to menstruation. Women susceptible to acne often report a worsening of the condition at this time.

Present evidence suggests that changes in eating habits, alterations in stress levels, and exposure to sunlight can make acne either better or worse. However, as the cause of acne is predominantly hormonal and hereditary, it is for the moment true to say that until it is possible to alter a person's genetic composition, acne will remain treatable, but not curable.

Black heads, white heads, and pimples are all caused, to varying degrees, by hyper-secretion of the sebaceous glands and associated infection.

In susceptible people, even slight exposure to many hair sprays may result in a sudden outbreak of acne. Plastic components in the spray block the larger pores, usually around the mouth, chin, and sides of the face, creating what is called an anaerobic (or "no air") environment. Many commonplace facial bacteria are low-oxygen organisms and actually thrive in such conditions. So, if you suffer from acne, read the labels on cosmetic and hair products carefully and avoid any that contain synthetic polymers, such as vinyl and other plastics.

CONVENTIONAL TREATMENT

The standard treatment consists of regular doses of antibiotics that simply help to prevent the germs in the small fatty lumps from multiplying.

In very severe cases, vitamin A derivatives have been successful in relieving the symptoms of acne, but often only after an initial worsening of the condition. Both oral and topical therapies are contraindicated for pregnant women. Topical therapy, using tretinoin, may cause skin irritation. Oral therapy, using isotretinoin, is associated with more serious side effects, including musculoskeletal pain, especially in the joints; hair and vision loss; severe dry skin; and depression. Generally, only a dermatologist will prescribe this form of therapy.

ALTERNATIVE TREATMENT

The best alternative to conventional treatments is the use of essential oils, which are not only antibacterial and anti-inflammatory but are also able to regulate the natural production of sebum. It is imperative to keep the skin clean and to resist the temptation to squeeze the black or white heads. Squeezing only causes further inflammation and scarring. For hydrosols, see page 45; for infusions, see page 30; for oils, see pages 34–44; for steaming, see page 33.

TWICE DAILY

to cleanse Apply a simple cleansing lotion, using 1 part witch hazel hydrosol, 1 part cold chamomile infusion, and a few drops of fresh lemon juice. This mix has a shelf life of seven days in a refrigerator, so make a week's supply at a time.

to control bacterial activity Massage the affected areas, combining an astringent carrier oil, such as hazelnut, with:

1. one of the antibacterial essential oils (niaouli, tea tree, or thyme) and
2. one of the anti-inflammatory oils (chamomile or lavender).

TWICE A WEEK

to deep cleanse and nourish Apply the revitalizing clay and spirulina recipe (see page 74). Apart from removing oil, dirt, and bacteria very effectively, the clay contains minerals (including oxide of iron, calcium, and various salts) and trace elements (including copper, magnesium, and zinc) that help the natural healing of damaged skin, while spirulina provides the whole spectrum of vitamin A. You can boost this mix by adding 3 drops of chamomile, niaouli, or thyme essential oil to the clay before the liquid. Alternatively, just add your essential oil to a simple clay mask (see page 23).

ONCE A WEEK OR MORE
to remove excess oil and open clogged pores Steam, adding a few drops of one of the anti-inflammatory or antibacterial essential oils listed above or 1 heaping tablespoon of dried herbs, such as chamomile, calendula, thyme, or yarrow. This will also help to eliminate redness.

boils

In most cases caused by a bacterial infection, boils are sited in hair follicles. A large, single boil or a tight group of smaller boils develops, with an accumulation of pus, swelling, inflammation, and pain.

CONVENTIONAL TREATMENT
A course of antibiotics is the usual prescription. Some scarring may occur, especially if (as often happens) boils reappear in the same place.

ALTERNATIVE TREATMENT
For oils, see pages 34–41; for clay, see pages 22–24; for infusions, see page 30.

DAILY
to reduce pain and inflammation Apply a slice (or the pulp) of a raw potato. Raw cabbage leaf is also very good for reducing inflammation and promoting healing.
to heal Apply undiluted niaouli or tea tree essential oil to the infected area, using cotton pads, three or four times a day.

WEEKLY

to deep cleanse A local application of a basic clay mix will help to eliminate pus, toxins, and residual infection. You may choose to substitute cucumber juice or a cold infusion of chamomile for the water.

AFTER HEALING

to reduce scarring and prevent further infection Using light massage twice daily, apply a mix of equal amounts of rosehip seed and sweet almond carrier oils, blended with 5 percent of two essential oils: niaouli and lavender or tea tree and lavender.

cracks and fissures

These often appear at the corners of the mouth, the edge of the nostrils, and behind the ears, less commonly on the fingers, and are sometimes complicated by fungal or bacterial infections.

CONVENTIONAL TREATMENT

Most people rely on an over-the-counter antiseptic cream.

ALTERNATIVE TREATMENT

For oils, see pages 34–41.

TWICE DAILY

to heal Apply an oil mix locally, combining apricot kernel and 10 percent vitamin E oil or half-and-half calendula and rosehip seed as the carrier, blended with a healing/astringent essential oil, such as cedarwood or cypress, and one of the following antiseptic essential oils: lavender, niaouli, or tea tree. An application of fresh, raw cabbage leaf may also be effective.

damaged skin

The general appearance of skin severely scarred by acne, accident, burns, or surgery or thickened as the result of chronic eczema can often be improved, using a natural skin care program. Conventional treatment is non-existent.

ALTERNATIVE TREATMENT

It is essential to cleanse damaged skin well before applying healing oils or masks. Clay masks are particularly useful, and the substitution of freshly pressed pineapple or papaya for water in a standard clay mask greatly increases the mask's action upon the epidermis. For oils, see pages 34–41; for clay, see pages 22–24.

DAILY

to reduce inflammation Vegetable masks are useful. Substitute a cabbage leaf in the lettuce-leaf treatment (see page 87) or simply dab on a half-and-half mix of fresh cabbage and carrot juices. Add a little clay powder to the juices as a thickening agent to make another simple mask. Leave it on the skin for 20 minutes before removing with bottled or spring water and cotton pads.

to improve appearance Using a cotton pad or your hands, apply one of the following oil mixes locally, to slightly dampened skin. The contents of three capsules of 500 I.U. borage or evening primrose and 400 I.U. vitamin E may also be added to either. Note: 20 drops of essential oil = ⅕ teaspoon (1ml).

1. Carrier oil: 3½ fl.oz. (100ml) rosehip seed. Essential oils: ⅕ teaspoon (1ml) cedarwood, ⅖ teaspoon (2ml) geranium, ⅕ teaspoon (1ml) rosewood, and ⅕ teaspoon (1ml) sandalwood.

2. Carrier oils: 2 fl.oz. (50ml) rosehip seed, 5 teaspoons (25ml) calendula, and 5 teaspoons (25ml) hypericum. Essential oils: ⅖ teaspoon (2ml) frankincense, ⅖ teaspoon (2ml) palmarosa, and ⅕ teaspoon (1ml) rosemary.

TWICE A WEEK

to deep cleanse Use a pineapple exfoliating mask (see page 65) or a papaya exfoliating lotion (see page 68). The application of undiluted papaya juice is a speedier alternative. Remove after 5 minutes.

eczema

This condition affects about one person in four. The symptomatic rash is accompanied by swelling, blistering, itching, and scaling. Bacteria tend to proliferate in the affected areas, causing the skin to become inflamed, infected, and sometimes weepy. Although eczema can be an allergic reaction, the causes are sometimes unknown. Some types of eczema are thought to be hereditary and are, therefore, difficult to treat.

CONVENTIONAL TREATMENT
A regimen of antibiotics, anti-inflammatories, and cortisone cream is the recommended approach.

ALTERNATIVE TREATMENT
For chronic eczema, consider also the treatment indicated in the section on damaged skin. For oils, see pages 34–41; for clay, see pages 22–24; for infusions, see page 30.

DAILY
to reduce inflammation See the section on damaged skin. Cucumber, potato, or watercress juice may also be applied directly to the skin with a cotton pad.

to soothe and heal Massage with an oil mix twice daily. The most useful essential oils are the anti-inflammatories, such as chamomile or lavender, and the antibacterial, anti-fungal, and antiviral oils, such as juniper, lemon, niaouli, rosewood, and tea tree. Choose two or three essential oils and mix with calendula, hypericum, or rosehip seed carrier oil. If the skin is very dry, substitute in the carrier oil(s) 10 percent each of one or two of the following: borage (or evening primrose oil) and vitamin E.

TWICE A WEEK
to soothe, cleanse, and heal Apply a clay mask, using fresh cucumber, carrot, cabbage, grape or melon juice, or an infusion of chamomile instead of water. If the skin is very dry, add 1 tablespoon of olive oil to the mask.

psoriasis

This chronic, hereditary skin condition is characterized by the accumulation of excessive numbers of cells in the epidermis that cause inflammation and flaking. Lengthy periods of remission are common.

CONVENTIONAL TREATMENT

Moderate cases are treated with preparations containing coal tar, salicylic acid or zinc, and psoralen, accompanied by ultraviolet radiation.

In the worst cases, the regular administration of oral or topical vitamin A derivatives may relieve symptoms. However, topical therapy, using tazarotene, irritates the skin, and oral therapy, using acetretin or soriatane, produces serious side effects similar to those produced by isotretinoin (see the section on acne). Oral therapy is rarely given to women of childbearing age.

ALTERNATIVE TREATMENT

The sun has a very beneficial effect on psoriatic skin. Daily massage with a mix of olive oil and the essential oil bergamot often produces improvement without significant side effects. Use no more than ⅕ teaspoon (1ml) of bergamot to 3½ fl.oz. (100ml) of olive oil. Bergamot is not listed in the essential oil chart because it contains a molecule called psoralene that renders the skin more sensitive to UVB rays (see page 9), making it unsuitable for more general use. For oils, see pages 34–39.

rosacea

At first, the sufferer exhibits a mass of tiny red spots on and around the nose and cheeks. Symptoms appear suddenly, accompanied by extreme itching or a burning sensation, and subside, and then the cycle begins again. At a late stage of chronic rosacea, congestion and even deformity in the affected area (especially of the nose) may occur. Skin affected by rosacea is dry, hot, and inflamed, but this condition is often associated with an oily condition of the skin, such as acne or seborrhoeic dermatitis. The cause is unknown.

CONVENTIONAL TREATMENT

The regular use of antibiotics is the most common therapy. In extreme cases, cosmetic surgery is the only option. Large amounts of the affected tissues of the nose and surrounding area are removed, which certainly improves the shape of the nose and the general appearance of the face, but it cannot be done without a certain amount of scarring.

ALTERNATIVE TREATMENT

Rosacea should be treated at the earliest possible stage to obtain the best results. Antibacterial and anti-inflammatory essential oils constitute the best alternative to conventional treatment and its long-term side effects. For oils, see pages 34–41; for infusions, see page 30; for clay, see pages 22–24.

DAILY

to heal and soothe Using an astringent carrier oil, such as hazelnut, combined with calendula or hypericum and a blend of two essential oils chosen from chamomile, geranium, lavender, palmarosa, rosewood, and tea tree, it is possible to regain control over the condition and often cure it. Apply with cotton pads, dabbing gently.

to soothe A chamomile infusion may bring quick relief from pain and inflammation. Cabbage, lettuce, and watercress are also good for acute inflammation. The cooked leaves can be applied directly to the skin (see page 87) or the juice mixed with an equal quantity of cucumber juice and used as a lotion or substituted for water in a basic clay mask. Alternatively, a purée can be mixed with an equal amount of clay powder, adjusting with more purée or clay (if necessary) for a simple mask.

TWICE A WEEK

to eliminate inflammation Regular application of a cooling clay mask using cucumber juice (see page 55) or a clay lotion, substituting a chamomile infusion for water (see page 58, VARIATION), is helpful. Do not steam the face.

to cool and soothe Melon and blackcurrant are anti-inflammatory. Use the fresh juice of either mixed with an infusion of chamomile as a calming, soothing lotion, and the pulp with clay as a mask (see "to soothe" on previous page).

seborrhoeic dermatitis

This inflammation is caused by hyperactive sebaceous glands (see page 6) and is most commonly found in people with oily or combination skin. It appears first on the forehead and sides of the nose, spreading rapidly to other parts of the face and the scalp. At this stage the sufferer looks sunburned and, indeed, often experiences a rather unpleasant, burning sensation. Fungal yeast organisms are always present in this type of inflammation.

CONVENTIONAL TREATMENT

Coal tar, zinc, and salicylic preparations are usually prescribed for the face and scalp. The condition also responds to antifungal preparations but is made considerably worse by the application of cortisone creams.

ALTERNATIVE TREATMENT

Antibacterial and anti-inflammatory essential oils that are able to regulate the production of sebum constitute the best alternative. For oils, see pages 34–44; for steaming, see page 33; for clay, see pages 22–24.

TWICE DAILY

to control bacterial or yeast activity Massage, using an astringent carrier oil, such as hazelnut, blended with one of the antifungal essential oils, such as niaouli, rosewood, or tea tree, and an anti-inflammatory oil, such as chamomile or lavender. Recent studies also indicate that the daily application of borage oil is rapidly beneficial in some cases. Apply locally, using a cotton pad, or supplement the carrier oil in the recipe above, using no more than 15 percent borage oil.

to soothe Cucumber juice and watercress or lettuce will calm acute inflammation. For watercress and lettuce, see the section on *rosacea*.

WEEKLY

to clean clogged pores Regular steaming will remove the excess sebum, and the addition of an anti-inflammatory and antibacterial oil or herb (see page 33) will help to eliminate some of the redness. Do this more than once a week, if possible.

to deep cleanse A basic clay mask is very effective. Apart from removing oils, dirt, and bacteria, clay can import minerals and trace elements valuable in the natural healing of damaged skin. The more powerful fruit masks, such as pineapple (see page 65) and papaya (see page 68), are also useful.

sunburn

If severe, see a doctor immediately or go to the nearest emergency room; you may require special dressings, antibiotics, or treatment for sunstroke.

ALTERNATIVE TREATMENT

For oils, see pages 34–41.

to soothe mild sunburn Dab undiluted lavender essential oil on the worst affected areas. On other areas, dilute the lavender oil in a half-and-half blend of calendula and olive oil carrier oils, using no more 5 percent lavender oil. Applications of raw cabbage or lettuce leaves are also helpful. Avoid masks of any kind.

Prevention, as always, is better than any cure, especially when you consider that prolonged exposure to the sun is the major cause of prematurely aged skin. For sun and the skin, see pages 8–11.

list of suppliers

All suppliers below offer mail-order services.

ATLANTIC SPICE CO.
PO Box 205
North Truro, MA 02652
tel: (800) 316-7965 (toll-free)
web: www.atlanticspice.com
*Oils, botanicals, and
miscellaneous supplies*

CAMDEN-GREY
ESSENTIAL OILS
7178-A SW 47 Street
Miami, FL 33155
tel: (877) 232-7662 (toll-free)
web: www.essentialoil.net
*Oils, hydrosols, packaging
materials, and books*

THE ESSENTIAL OIL
COMPANY
1719 SE Umatilla Street
Portland, OR 97202

tel: (800) 729-5912 (toll-free)
web: essentialoil.com/index2.html
Oils, hydrosols, and glassware

LEYDET AROMATICS
PO Box 2354
Fair Oaks, CA 95628
tel: (916) 965-7546
or (916) 962-3292
web: www.leydet.com
*Oils, hydrosols, and
educational resources*

LIBERTY NATURAL
PRODUCTS
8120 SE Stark Street
Portland, OR 97215
tel: (800)-289-8427 (toll-free)
web: www.libertynatural.com
*Bulk ingredients, massage
items, packaging containers,
books, and music*

MOUNTAIN ROSE
HERBS
20818 High Street
North San Juan, CA 95960
tel: (800) 879-3337 (toll-free)
web: www.mountainroseherbs.com
*Oils, herbs, hydrosols, bottles
and jars, and books*

NEAL'S YARD REMEDIES
79 East Putnam Avenue
Greenwich, CT 06830
tel: (888) 697-8721 (toll-free)
web: www.nyr-usa.com
*Oils, skin and hair care guides,
herbs, and related publications*

SAMARA BOTANE
1811 Queen Anne Avenue
N. Ste 103
Seattle, WA 98109
tel: (800) 782-4532 (toll-free)

or (206) 283-7191 (shop)
web: www.wingedseed.com
*Oils, hydrosols, distillation
equipment, books, and
accessories*

SUNBURST BOTTLE
COMPANY
5710 Auburn Boulevard Ste
7, Sacramento, CA 95841
tel: (916) 348-5576
web: www.sunburstbottle.com
*Bottles of various shapes
and sizes*

index

128   anti-wrinkle treatments for perfect skin

ACKNOWLEDGMENTS

The photographs of all recipe ingredients were taken by Diana Miller and styled by Wei Tang. All other photographs, of massage and masks, were taken by Graham Atkins Hughes, and the masks and massage movements were modeled by Flavia Eberhard.

Publisher's Note

Please note that although this book includes recommended treatments for particular skin conditions, they are not substitutes for regular medication and treatment. We recommend that you consult your doctor before trying any of the treatments. While every care has been taken in compiling this book, no responsibility can be accepted by the author or the publishers for any consequence resulting directly or indirectly from the use or adaptation of any of the contents of this book, or from any omission from it.

The mission of Storey Communications is to serve our customers by publishing practical information that encourages personal independence in harmony with the environment.

United States edition published in 2001 by Storey Books, Schoolhouse Road, Pownal, Vermont 05261

First published in 2001 by Quadrille Publishing London WC2H OLS

© Text Pierre Jean Cousin 2001
© Design and layout Quadrille Publishing Limited 2001

Publishing Director: Anne Furniss
Consultant Art Director: Helen Lewis
Design Assistants: Sarah Emery and Katy Davis
Project Editor: Nicki Marshall
Editor: Mary Davies
Production: Sarah Tucker

Professional Assistance: Donna Maria

The information in this book is true and complete to the best of our knowledge. All recommendations are made without guarantee on the part of the author or Storey Books. The author and publisher disclaim any liability in connection with the use of this information. For additional information please contact Storey Books, Schoolhouse Road, Pownal, Vermont 05261.

Library of Congress Cataloging-in-Publication Data

Cousin, Pierre Jean.
Anti-wrinkle treatments for perfect skin: 48 recipes for masks, cleansers, toners, & lotions using fruit, herbs, honey & other nourishing ingredients / by Pierre Jean Cousin.

p. cm.
ISBN 1-58017-368-3 (alk. paper)

1. Beauty, Personal. 2. Face—Care and hygiene.
3. Women—Health and hygiene. 4. Cookery. I. Title.

RA776.5 .C6825 2001
646.7'26—dc21
00-050525

Printed and bound by Dai Nippon Printing, Hong Kong